Diabetes
For Canadians
FOR
DUMMIES®
SPECIAL EDITION

Diabetes
For Canadians
FOR
DUMMIES®
SPECIAL EDITION

by Alan L. Rubin, M.D.
Ian Blumer, M.D., F.R.C.P.(C)

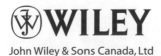

WILEY

John Wiley & Sons Canada, Ltd

Diabetes For Canadians For Dummies®

Published by
John Wiley & Sons Canada, Ltd
6045 Freemont Boulevard
Mississauga, Ontario, L5R 4J3
www.wiley.ca

For details on how to create a custom book for your company or organization, or for more information on John Wiley & Sons Canada custom publishing programs, please call 416 646-7992 or e-mail us at cupubcan@wiley.com

Diabetes For Canadians For Dummies / Ian Blumer.

ISBN: 0-470-83634-2

Printed in Canada

Distributed in Canada by John Wiley & Sons Canada, Ltd.

For general information on John Wiley & Sons Canada, Ltd., including all books published by Wiley Publishing, Inc., please call our warehouse, Tel 1-800-567-4797. For reseller information, including discounts and premium sales, please call our sales department, Tel 416-646-7992. For press review copies, author interviews, or other publicity information, please contact our marketing department, Tel: 416-646-4584, Fax 416-236-4448.

For authorization to photocopy items for corporate, personal, or educational use, please contact The Canadian Copyright Licensing Agency (Access Copyright). For an Access Copyright license, visit www.accesscopyright.ca or call toll free 1-800-893-5777.

About the Authors

Ian Blumer, M.D., F.R.C.P.(C), is a diabetes specialist with a community practice in the Durham region of Ontario. He has a teaching appointment as a medical associate with Mount Sinai Hospital (part of the University of Toronto) and is actively involved in diabetes research. An enthusiastic lecturer, he has spoken about diabetes to numerous professional and lay audiences and has appeared regularly in the Canadian media. He is a member of the Clinical and Scientific Section of the Canadian Diabetes Association, the American Diabetes Association, and the European Association for the Study of Diabetes. Ian is the author of *What Your Doctor Really Thinks* (Dundurn, 1999) and the medical advisor for the *Everything Diabetes Book* (Adams Media, 2003). His popular Web site (www.ianblumer.com) offers practical advice on how to manage diabetes. Ian is married to a rheumatologist and has three children, the eldest of which, to Ian's astonishment, is now old enough that she is attending university. In his spare time, Ian can be found skiing down mogul runs and battling wind and waves during a sailing race. One day he hopes to emulate lucky Vancouverites who get to do both on the same day, though not necessarily at the same time. Ian welcomes your comments about this book at diabetes@ianblumer.com.

Alan L. Rubin, M.D., is a professional member of the American Diabetes Association and the Endocrine Society and has been in private practice specializing in diabetes and thyroid disease for more than 28 years. Dr. Rubin was Assistant Clinical Professor of Medicine at University of California Medical Center in San Francisco for 20 years. He has spoken about diabetes to professional medical audiences and non-medical audiences around the world. He has been a consultant to many pharmaceutical companies and companies that make diabetes products.

Dedication

This book is dedicated to Ian's parents, Rhoda and Jack, whose love, generosity, and wisdom are as cherished today as they were way back when.

This book is also dedicated to Alan's wife, Enid, and to Alan's children, Renee and Larry. Their patience, enthusiasm, and encouragement helped to make Alan's writing a real pleasure.

Acknowledgements

Ian Blumer would like to let his wonderful wife, Heather, know that now this book is completed, he promises to once again spend leisurely Sunday breakfasts with her instead of with his laptop.

Ian would like to express his appreciation to Marian Barltrop, a superb diabetes educator and his research assistant on this project. Without her immensely helpful footwork, Ian would still be writing Chapter 1. Ian would also like to thank Bin Chin, a terrific dietitian and Ian's nutrition teacher, for her invaluable help with the Food Groups Appendix. Thanks also to the dietitians from across Canada that contributed recipes to the book. Marlene Grass, R.N., the epitome of selfless dedication and a pioneer in childhood and young adult diabetes education, cannot be thanked enough, not only for her helpful suggestions but moreover for her guidance by way of example. Drs. Amir Hanna, Stewart Harris, Ralph Kern, and Bernard Zinman are all to be thanked for their helpful tips. A special thanks to Dr. Anne Kenshole for her keen insights and thoughtful suggestions. Randall McDonald (Omni Insurance) and Wayne Redford (Allstate) were kind enough to provide assurance about insurance. Jeff Hirst, BPHE, PFLC, a former Canadian Olympian who is now a fitness consultant (Training Zone Inc.), has been an invaluable resource in all matters relating to the role of exercise in good diabetes health. Thanks, Jeff.

To all the nurse educators and dietitians in Durham and Northumberland counties that have worked with Ian over the past 20 years, thanks for your tireless efforts. Your unwavering commitment to the patients we serve is a constant reminder of the importance and value of working as a diabetes health care team. Ian hopes this book carries that message to all who read it.

Not a day goes by that Ian does not marvel at the skills of his greatest mentor, Dr. Barney Berris. Dr. Berris, "a physician's physician," is the epitome of all that is admirable in a doctor. Ian's choice of a career in internal medicine is in no small measure a result of the example set by this fine man.

Ian would like to thank his colleague, Alan Rubin, whose book, *Diabetes For Dummies,* created a wonderful foundation upon which this book could be created.

One group of teachers — our patients — deserves special attention. Their trials and tribulations have been our raison d'être.

Lastly, Ian wishes to thank Lisa Berland and Allyson Latta, whose skillful editing of this book has reminded Ian why he should have paid much more attention to his English teachers and much less attention to the Habs.

Alan Rubin thanks the great acquisitions editor and midwife, Tami Booth; she deserves great appreciation for helping to deliver this new baby. Her optimism and her ideas actually made this book possible. Alan's project editor, Kelly Ewing, has made sure that this book follows the laws of grammar and is readable and understandable in the great *For Dummies* tradition. Thanks to Dr. Seymour Levin for the technical editing of this book.

Dietitian Nancy Bennett evaluated all the recipes in the original edition, cooked them, tasted them, and put them into a form that readers could follow. She also provided great food for thought about the role of the dietitian in diabetes care.

Alan wants to thank ophthalmologist Dr. John Norris of Pacific Eye Associates in San Francisco for helping him to see the place of the eye physician in diabetes care. He also wants to thank podiatrist Dr. Mark Pinter for helping him get a leg up on his specialty.

Librarians Mary Ann Zaremska and Nancy Phelps at St. Francis Memorial Hospital were tremendously helpful in providing the articles and books upon which the information in the book is based.

Alan wants to thank Dr. Richard Bernstein of Marin County, California, for the many years of learning, collaboration, and enjoyment together.

Ronnie and Michael Goldfield should definitely be considered the godparents of this book.

Alan's friends in the Dawn Patrol kept him laughing through-out the production of this book. Their willingness to follow him convinced him that others would be willing to read what he wrote.

Alan's teachers are too numerous to mention, but one group deserves special attention. They are his patients over the last 28 years, the people whose trials and tribulations caused him to seek the knowledge that you will find in this book.

This book is written on the shoulders of thousands of men and women who made the discoveries and held the committee meetings. Their accomplishments cannot possibly be given adequate acclaim. We owe them big time.

Publisher's Acknowledgements

We're proud of this book; please send us your comments at canadapt@wiley.com. Some of the people who helped bring this book to market include the following:

Acquisitions and Editorial

Associate Editor: Robert Hickey

Developmental Editor: Lisa Berland

Copy Editor: Allyson Latta

Manager, Custom Publishing:
Christiane Coté

Production

Publishing Services Director:
Karen Bryan

Publishing Services Manager: Ian Koo

Project Manager: Elizabeth McCurdy

Project Coordinator: Pam Vokey

Layout and Graphics: Pat Loi

Proofreader: Susan Gaines

John Wiley & Sons Canada, Ltd.

Bill Zerter, Chief Operating Officer

Robert Harris, General Manager, Professional and Trade Division

Publishing and Editorial for Consumer Dummies

Diane Graves Steele, Vice President and Publisher, Consumer Dummies

Joyce Pepple, Acquisitions Director, Consumer Dummies

Kristin A. Cocks, Product Development Director, Consumer Dummies

Michael Spring, Vice President and Publisher, Travel

Suzanne Jannetta, Editorial Director, Travel

Publishing for Technology Dummies

Andy Cummings, Acquisitions Director

Composition Services

Gerry Fahey, Executive Director of Production Services

Debbie Stailey, Director of Composition Services

Table of Contents

Introduction

*I*s there ever a good time to have diabetes? No, of course there isn't. But at the beginning of the 21st century, people with diabetes are better off than at any other time in history. A hundred years ago, people with diabetes did not live very long. As recently as 30 years ago, most people with diabetes were destined to suffer all sorts of complications often including blindness and amputations. But now we have the means to protect ourselves. We can lead not only long lives, but full, active, and healthy lives. And it all starts with knowledge. Because when it comes to diabetes, knowledge is power and the key to success.

About This Book

This special abridged edition of *Diabetes For Canadians For Dummies* is not meant to be read from cover to cover, although if you know nothing about diabetes, it might be a good approach to do so. This book is to serve as a source for information about diabetes, what causes it, how it affects you, and, most importantly, how to effectively deal with diabetes so that you can achieve and maintain good health.

Canada has a long and proud history of being in the forefront of diabetes research and therapy. *Diabetes For Canadians For Dummies* looks at the special issues that Canadians with diabetes have to face (like Ian's patient who returned to his car one February morning after his son's hockey practice, only to find his insulin frozen solid!) and uses the most recent Canadian Diabetes Association recommendations ("2003 Clinical Practice Guidelines for the Prevention and Management of Diabetes in Canada").

In addition to discussing the latest facts about diabetes, this book tells you about the best sources you can access to discover any information that comes out after the publication of this edition. You will find frequent reference to Web sites that offer excellent information. If you do not have Internet access yourself, you can still get online at your neighbourhood library. As Internet addresses change frequently, we generally will refer to the "home page" of a site, from where you can follow the links to the appropriate Web page.

As you may have already noticed, this book was co-written by Ian (that would be me) and Alan (that would be me). Fortunately, we share the same perspectives on diabetes management. (Thank goodness! Sure would have been hard to write this book otherwise.)

Conventions Used in This Book

Diabetes, as you know, is associated with sugar problems. But sugars come in many types, so doctors avoid using the words *sugar* and *glucose* interchangeably. In this book (unless we slip up), we use the word *glucose* rather than *sugar*. As well, because it gets to be redundant to keep adding *mmol/L* after every blood glucose value to which we refer, you can safely assume that when we say, for example, that a normal fasting blood glucose is under 6.1, we mean 6.1 *mmol/L*.

Icons Used in This Book

The icons tell you what you must know, what you should know, and what you might find interesting but can live without.

This icon indicates a story about one of our patients.

This icon marks paragraphs where we define terms.

When you see this icon, it means the information is critical and is not to be missed.

This icon points out when you should contact your health care team (for example, if your blood glucose control is in need of improving or if you need a particular test done). Your health care team includes your family doctor, your diabetes specialist, your diabetes educator, your dietitian, your eye doctor, your pharmacist, and, when necessary, other specialists (such as a podiatrist, dentist, cardiologist, kidney specialist, neurologist, emergency room physician, and so forth). We will let you know which member of your team you should contact. (Incidentally, the most important member of your health care team is you.)

 This icon is used when we share a practical, time-saving piece of advice, sometimes providing some additional detail on an important point.

Chapter 1

Membership in a Club You Didn't Ask to Join

*A*s a person with diabetes, you already know that diabetes isn't "just a glucose problem." In fact, the moment you were told you had diabetes, many different thoughts may have run through your mind. You have feelings, and you have your own personal story. You are not the same person as your next-door neighbour or your sister or your friend, and your diabetes and the way that you respond to its challenges are unique to you.

This chapter gives you a quick definition of diabetes and tells you about some celebrated folks who have diabetes, too.

What Is Diabetes?

Since we are going to be spending so much time discussing diabetes, let's start by defining the condition. That should be a simple enough task — except that many dictionaries (including, sorry to say, Canadian ones) define it incorrectly. The simplest, *correct* definition is that diabetes is a disease in which there is too much glucose in the blood due to insufficient or ineffective insulin. Although that is technically correct, it misses out on so, so much, because diabetes is not just a problem of glucose; it is a *whole* body problem. To make this point, Ian has had a burst of creativity and has gone ahead and made up his own definition of diabetes: "a disease in which there are high blood glucose levels *and* an increased risk of damage to the body, much of which is preventable."

"Diabetes" is actually the short form for *diabetes mellitus*. The Romans had noticed that the urine of certain people was *mellitus*, the Latin word for *sweet*. The Greeks noticed that when people with sweet urine drank, fluids came out in the urine almost as fast as they went in the mouth, like a siphon. They called this by the Greek word for *siphon* — diabetes. Hence, diabetes mellitus, but we think this is much better captured by the 17th-century definition of diabetes: "the pissing evil." Talk about calling it the way you see it!

You Are Not Alone

Ian remembers encountering a huge lineup in front of one particular exhibit while attending a diabetes conference a few years back. There were so many people in line, in fact, that he figured there must have been some amazing new breakthrough product being demonstrated. Well, as it turns out, the big attraction was actually Nicole Johnson, the 1999 Miss America. She was there to talk about how she managed her diabetes.

Perhaps you have seen a movie starring the Academy-award winning actress Halle Berry. It's not likely that you noticed her diabetes affecting her acting, or her beauty for that matter. Similarly, you likely did not notice diabetes preventing the great success of athletes like Bobbie Clarke, Jackie Robinson or golf star Scott Verplank, authors like Ernest Hemingway or H. G. Wells, musicians like B. B. King and Jerry Garcia (of the Grateful Dead — which came long before Cherry Garcia ice cream!) or inventors like Thomas Edison, to name but a few famous people with diabetes.

John Dennis is a Canadian who likes to sail. That he also has diabetes does not make him unique in the sailing community. Oh, did we happen to mention where he sails? That would be circumnavigating the globe. Alone!

You may not have spoken to Stephen Steele, but it is quite possible he has spoken to you. Stephen is a commercial pilot with a major Canadian airline. And in the event that you have the bad luck to be in dire straits on some sinking vessel off the Atlantic coast, it is quite possible that the hero plucking you from the ocean will be none other than Major Chuck Grenkow, a Medal of Bravery–winning Canadian Forces pilot and aircraft commander performing search and rescue operations with the Canadian military. Oh, by the way, they both have insulin-treated diabetes.

Diabetes is a common disease, so it's bound to occur in some very uncommon people. Have a look at the Famous Diabetics Web site (www.angelarose.com/FamousDiabetics/index.html). But one does not have to be famous to be considered exceptional. Indeed, every day of the week we see special people, people who have diabetes yet look after families, work in automotive plants or office buildings, write exams, go to movies, and do their best to live life to the fullest. People just like you.

The point is, diabetes should not define your life. You are the same person the day after you found out you had diabetes as you were the day before. It just happens that you have been given an additional issue to deal with. Diabetes should not stop you from doing what you want to do with your life. Certainly, it does complicate things in some ways, but if you follow the rules of good diabetes care that are discussed in this book, you may actually be *healthier* than people without diabetes who smoke, overeat, under-exercise, or engage in other, unhealthy activities.

Chapter 2

Glucose and You

● ●

● ●

*T*he ancient Greeks and Romans knew about diabetes. Fortunately, the way they tested for the condition — by tasting the urine — has gone by the wayside.

Most people with diabetes are diagnosed when they have their blood glucose level measured either as part of a routine check-up with their family doctor, or for some other coincidental reason (such as at the time of an insurance application or in preparation for surgery). Occasionally, a person with diabetes has the condition diagnosed after they develop symptoms that they recognize may be due to high blood glucose and they see their doctor asking to be tested for this.

Ian recently saw a 50-year-old businessman in the office. He had started to get up during the night to pass his urine. At first he blamed it on his prostate, but when he noticed that he was unexpectedly losing weight he recalled that a close relative had experienced similar symptoms and had been found to have diabetes. The businessman decided he should be tested for this too. His blood glucose turned out to be two times higher than normal. Ian had him meet up with a dietitian and a diabetes educator, and, with proper lifestyle measures, his glucose level was down to normal in a matter of weeks. He finally started to get a good night's sleep again, his energy improved, and his business took off. Now, his competitors may not have been too happy, but that's a different story.

You may have done some searching in books or on the Internet and come across another form of diabetes called *diabetes insipidus*. This term refers to an *entirely* different condition than diabetes mellitus. The only thing they have in common is a tendency to pass lots of urine. And now that we've clarified that, you will not see diabetes insipidus mentioned again in this book.

What Is Glucose?

The sweetness of the urine with which the ancients had first-hand experience comes from *glucose*, also known as blood *sugar*. There are many different kinds of sugar, but the important one when it comes to diabetes is glucose. Glucose is the fuel that your body uses to provide instant energy so that muscles can move and important chemical reactions can take place. Sugar is a carbohydrate, one group of the three sources of energy in the body. The others are protein and fat, which we discuss in greater detail in Chapter 7.

Unlike in high school chemistry class, here we are going to let you off easy and, apart from our discussion about nutrition therapy, we won't talk about all the other sugars that are around. But just in case you are wondering, some examples of other sugars are fructose (the sugar found in fruits and vegetables) and sucrose (actually a combination of glucose and fructose).

How Diabetes Is Diagnosed

Diagnosing diabetes should be simple. You know by now that you have diabetes when your glucose level is too high. But what, exactly, is too high? One way to think of "too high" is to think of the level of blood glucose that can cause damage to your body. More difficult is attaching a specific number to that level. Different countries have different ways of deciding that, but in Canada we consider someone to have diabetes if they meet *any* one of the following three criteria:

- ✔ A **casual** blood glucose level ("casual" is defined as any time of day or night, without regard to the interval since the last time you ingested anything containing calories) equal to or greater than 11.1 millimoles per litre (mmol/L) with symptoms of high blood glucose (we discuss these symptoms in the next section).

- ✔ A **fasting** blood glucose level ("fasting" is defined as 8 or more hours without calorie intake) equal to or greater than 7.0 mmol/L.

- ✔ A blood glucose level equal to or greater than 11.1 mmol/L, when tested 2 hours after ingesting 75 grams of glucose as part of what is called a "**glucose tolerance test.**" Doctors used to order this test quite often, but nowadays doctors have learned that it is usually unnecessary. The diagnosis of diabetes can generally be made more easily with one of the other two tests we just mentioned.

Testing positive for one of the above criteria is not enough to result in a diagnosis of diabetes. Any one of the tests must be positive on *another* day to establish the diagnosis. More than one patient has come to us with a diagnosis of diabetes after having been tested only once, and then when we retested their blood glucose it turned out to be normal. They didn't have diabetes after all. Remember that the diagnosis of diabetes should be based on a blood sample taken from a *vein*. If you borrow your friend's glucose meter (which you shouldn't do by the way; as we discuss in Chapter 6) and find your glucose level to be high, see your doctor to have a blood sample drawn at a laboratory. Don't diagnose yourself based on a glucose meter result.

The only time that a diagnosis of diabetes can be made without repeating a blood glucose test is if your blood glucose level is very high and you are clearly ill from it.

If you have visited U.S. Web sites you may have noticed that there (and nowhere else) they use different units — called milligrams per decilitre (abbreviated mg/dL). To convert mg/dL to mmol/L you divide mg/dL by 18: for example 200 mg/dL divided by 18 equals 11.1 mmol/L. And we promise that will be the last time we *ever* mention how they measure blood glucose outside of Canada!

Controlling Glucose

Although there may never be a *good* time to have diabetes, far better to have it now than 100 years ago, when almost no therapy was available. Until insulin was discovered in the 1920s, little could be done to help people with diabetes. For years after that, insulin was the mainstay of therapy, but in the middle years of the last century a number of different drugs were discovered that combat high blood glucose (hyperglycemia). And in the later years of the 20th century, further discoveries made several entirely new types of medicine available. As Ian likes to say, it was about time that diabetes specialists were given more tools; we were getting very jealous of cardiologists who seemed to be getting all the neat drugs. Nowadays virtually anyone with diabetes can have excellent blood glucose control. It may not always be easy to achieve, but it *can* be achieved and, indeed, *must* be achieved if you are going to keep healthy.

Treatment is not just a matter of taking medicine, of course. In fact, medicine is often the least important of the diabetes treatments. The three key therapies are:

- Diet (more aptly called nutrition therapy; see Chapter 7)
- Exercise
- Medication

Most people with diabetes require a combination of all three of these strategies.

Losing Control of Glucose

You will find that once you improve your blood glucose control, you will feel better. You won't be running to the bathroom around the clock, your energy level will improve, and you will have a better sense of well-being. There will be times, however, when your blood glucose control worsens and some of your symptoms may start to return. You may find that things worsen if you are under greater stress, or if you have gotten off track with your nutrition plan, or if there has been yet another February blizzard and the idea of going out for your daily walk is just too daunting.

There are two main things to remember when your glucose control worsens:

✔ If you are feeling reasonably well, then even if your blood glucose levels climb up into the high teens (or even somewhat higher) there is no immediate danger to you. (The exception to this is if you have type 1 diabetes and are developing ketones. See Chapter 4 for a discussion of ketoacidosis). A few days of blood glucose readings of 20 will not damage your organs.

✔ Take it as a message that something is wrong and take corrective action. This may be as simple as adjusting your diet or restarting your exercise plan. Perhaps you have simply forgotten to refill a prescription for your oral hypoglycemic agent, in which case a trip to the pharmacy is in order.

If your blood glucose readings have risen to the high teens or higher and you are feeling unwell (or if you have type 1 diabetes and you have developed ketones), then you need to seek immediate medical assistance. If you are very ill, proceed to the nearest emergency department. If you are not feeling all that badly, you may first contact your physician. (Some diabetes educators are trained and empowered to assist you with these situations also.)

Diabetes in Canada

Diabetes is a serious health problem, both for the individual with diabetes and for society as a whole. In Canada, there are more than 2 million people with diabetes (many of whom are not diagnosed). The older you get the more likely you are to have diabetes — some estimates suggest that as many as one out of every five people over the age of 60 in Canada has diabetes.

Canada is not unique in this realm. Indeed, virtually every country is experiencing alarming growth rates of diabetes and it is estimated that by the year 2010 there will be 300 million people world-wide with diabetes. Researchers once believed that the increasing numbers were a result of the advancing average age of the population, but recent evidence suggests that it may simply be the result of the fact that as we get older we tend to become overweight. Thus it may not be aging in itself that makes us more likely to get diabetes. (The

(continued)

(continued)

moral: Eat properly and exercise whether you are 2 or 82.)

Interestingly, Japanese Sumo wrestlers — not exactly lightweights — have an extraordinarily high likelihood of getting diabetes. And it's even greater once they retire — as high as 40 percent!

The yearly economic costs of diabetes in Canada are estimated to be a staggering $12 billion. That is not a misprint. That's $12 billion! That works out to an average of $6,000 for every man, woman, and child with diabetes and even at that likely represents an underestimate. Can you just imagine the ways you could spend that money?

As a diabetes specialist practising in Canada, Ian has been terribly frustrated by the lack of attention that governments and hospital administrators have traditionally paid to diabetes. Diabetes is not a dramatic illness like heart disease. Diabetes usually does not draw on the emotional purse strings in the way that cancer (appropriately) does. And diabetes does not have the aura of glamour and mystique that surrounds complex procedures such as brain or heart surgery. Many people even think that with insulin and other therapies, diabetes is "just an inconvenience." Surely these people do not have diabetes themselves.

There has long been a tendency amongst health care policy-makers to address what are sometimes cynically called "sexy" problems, including the illnesses just mentioned. Diabetes simply hasn't been on the radar screen. Indeed, hospital administrators have reduced staff at diabetes education centres as they try to deal with their own fiscal restraints. Diabetes education is considered expendable because administrators and bureaucrats do not see short-term return on their economic investments. And that is a tragedy, because money spent on diabetes education would come back a hundredfold in savings, preventing complications and thus keeping people with diabetes healthy (and out of hospital!).

Thankfully, governments in Canada are finally coming to grips with the need to improve diabetes services and, in particular, working toward initiating preventive strategies. Hospitals are still lagging behind, though, and we can only hope that, working in concert with government and with the encouragement (read "pressure") of people like you and physicians like us, hospitals will not only stop cutting back on diabetes services but enhance them. Even better, let's get diabetes education centres out of hospitals and into the communities where they belong!

For a further discussion about the health care costs of diabetes in Canada, have a look at *Diabetes in Canada,* Second Edition, issued by Health Canada (www.hc-sc.gc.ca/pphb-dgspsp/publicat/dic-dac2/english/01cover_e.html).

Chapter 3

What Type of Diabetes Do You Have?

*Y*ou might think that diabetes is diabetes is diabetes. And, true enough, in many ways the various forms of diabetes have much in common. Everyone with diabetes is combating a tendency to have high blood glucose levels and everyone with diabetes has to make appropriate dietary changes to enhance their health. And whether you are age 5 or 95, it is essential that you have proper eye care, proper foot care, and all the other things that go along with achieving and maintaining good health.

Having said that, there are certain things that are unique to the different forms of diabetes and that require special attention. In this chapter we look at these different forms of diabetes, determining what they have in common and how they differ.

 Jim Tucker, a 50-year-old assembly-line worker at a car plant, had always been the picture of health. Indeed, he never saw doctors. He was a hard-working man who enjoyed spending time playing ball in the summer and hockey in the winter. Over the past few months he had noticed that he was going to the bathroom night and day. And he was constantly thirsty.

Thinking that he needed better nutrition he had started to drink glass after glass of orange juice. But that didn't make him feel better. One day he got on the scale and realized that, although he was still overweight, during the past six months he had lost fifteen pounds without even trying. Jim was hesitant to see a doctor, but his wife finally convinced him that he had to get checked out. He went to see his family physician, a blood test was done, and a day later Jim got a call at work that he had to come in to see the doctor right away. His blood glucose level was 25. Jim's doctor told him the result and what it meant. Jim had *type 2 diabetes*.

Mary was a 5-year-old girl. She was a beautiful, healthy, and happy child, but had suddenly become irritable and in just a matter of days had started to look increasingly unwell. She was quickly losing weight and had started to wet her bed. Mary's parents became alarmed and took her to the local emergency department, where doctors found that she had a blood glucose level of 15 and that her urine contained a substance called ketones. Mary was diagnosed as having *type 1 diabetes*.

What do Jim and Mary have in common? That is easy to answer and takes but one word: *diabetes*. But if we were to write about how they *differ*, that would take a whole chapter. This chapter . . .

You Have Type 1 Diabetes

Until just a few years ago, the way that diabetes was classified was very different (and very confusing!). What we now refer to as type 1 diabetes used to be called "juvenile-onset diabetes" or "insulin dependent diabetes." And what we now call type 2 diabetes used to be called "adult-onset diabetes" or "non-insulin dependent diabetes."

The problem with the old terms is that many people don't fit the descriptive titles. For example, many children who get diabetes actually have type 2 diabetes. And many adults who get diabetes actually have type 1 diabetes. So if we had stuck with the old terms we would be telling tons of kids they have "adult-onset diabetes" and tons of adults they have "juvenile-onset diabetes." Now, in our books, even if you have got a thick head of jet-black hair, a "six-pack" muscled belly, and nary a wrinkle on your perfect skin, it still doesn't seem right to say that you have a "juvenile" disease if you are 40 years old. And telling a 10-year-old that he or she has an "adult" disease doesn't seem sensible either.

Unfortunately, you are still likely to come across the outdated names because many people — including some health care providers — haven't caught up yet with the new terminology.

You can have type 2 diabetes and require insulin, but that does *not* mean you now have type 1 diabetes. You still have type 2 diabetes even though you require insulin therapy.

Identifying the symptoms of type 1 diabetes

Type 1 diabetes almost always gets discovered *before it* has caused any irreversible damage to your body. Why? Because once type 1 diabetes has developed, symptoms tend to come on quite quickly. Symptoms include the following:

- **Frequent urination:** Passing lots of urine is a typical symptom of diabetes. You experience frequent urination because once your blood glucose level rises to above 10 or so (people without diabetes seldom have values above 8), glucose passes through the kidneys and spills into the urine, drawing extra fluids along the way.

- **Increase in thirst:** Because you are losing excess fluids in the urine, you are at risk of getting dehydrated. Your clever body tries to prevent this by making you feel thirstier, which, of course, encourages you to drink more.

- **Weight loss and increased hunger:** It is no coincidence that long, long ago, if someone was suspected as having diabetes, their urine was placed near an anthill to see if the little critters would be attracted to it. They knew dinner when they smelled it. If you have (uncontrolled) type 1 diabetes, you are passing urine that is rich in glucose and, thus, is rich in calories. This wasted nutrition is going down the drain in a manner of speaking. The body then starts to break down muscle and fat tissue. Your body doesn't like that one bit, so it makes you hungry, hoping that that will encourage you to eat more to maintain your health.

✔ **Fatigue:** When type 1 diabetes first strikes, you suddenly start to lose body fluids, muscle mass, and fat tissue, and you quickly become malnourished and are on the verge of being (or actually are) dehydrated. In the face of this onslaught, it is no wonder you feel fatigued. If you have type 1 diabetes, you probably recall how quickly your energy improved once you started insulin therapy.

✔ **Fruity breath:** When your body cannot use glucose as a fuel, it looks for alternative sources of energy, one of which is fat tissue. As fat tissue breaks down, it releases acids called ketones and these typically make the breath smell fruity, very much like a candy mint. If lots of ketones are present this can be a sign of a dangerous condition called *ketoacidosis*, which we discuss further in Chapter 4.

✔ **Blurred vision:** When the glucose levels in your body undergo a big change, the fluid content of the lens of your eyes also changes. That, in turn, alters the way that light bends as it passes through your eyes and leads to blurring. Maybe you have noticed the way that a knife in a glass of water looks bent. It is much the same phenomenon.

Investigating the causes of type 1 diabetes

If you or someone you love has type 1 diabetes, after you get over the shock of hearing the news, the next thing you will probably ask is "How could this have happened?" And that is an excellent question. In fact that is the same question scientists have been asking for many, many years, and it still goes unanswered.

We *do* know that type 1 diabetes is not contagious and you can rest assured that you did not get it from someone with diabetes sneezing on you or coughing on you. And you did not get type 1 diabetes from eating the wrong foods or not exercising enough or from being under stress. In fact, you did nothing wrong at all. Type 1 diabetes is *not* something that you brought on; it is something that happened to you.

Type 1 diabetes is an *autoimmune disease*, meaning that your body has been unkind enough to react against itself. There are many different types of autoimmune disease, including certain types of thyroid disease and arthritis conditions such as lupus and rheumatoid arthritis.

We all make antibodies to fight off infections, but in the case of type 1 diabetes your body creates antibodies that have decided that your own insulin-producing, islet cells of your pancreas are the enemy and have attacked these cells. This can be demonstrated by checking for certain antibodies in the blood stream, including islet cell antibodies, insulin antibodies, and GAD (*glutamic acid decarboxylase*) antibodies. It is seldom necessary to test for these antibodies outside of research settings (and in Canada the cost for these tests is usually not covered by health insurance plans — another strong disincentive to ordering them).

We don't know why your immune system would turn against your pancreas, but there are a number of theories:

- ✔ At various times in our lives we develop viral infections and our bodies fight these off by producing antibodies. It could be that one of these viruses shared something in its appearance with an islet cell and the body's antibodies couldn't separate out the good guys (your islet cells) from the bad guys (the virus) and attacked both.

- ✔ Non-breastfed babies have a higher risk of developing type 1 diabetes. It could be that a protein in cows' milk causes the same sort of response as a virus and, just as we discussed in the preceding paragraph, leads to an antibody attack on your own pancreas. This possibility is being looked at in the TRIGR study (*T*rial to *R*educe *I*DDM in the *G*enetically at *R*isk; www.trigr.org). This study looks at the risk of developing diabetes in babies who, if they are unable to breastfeed, are given one of 2 types of formula; either a standard, cow's milk based formula or a formula that is made up of smaller, less complex proteins that will possibly be less likely to stimulate an inappropriate immune system response (which, in turn, may reduce the likelihood of diabetes).

- ✔ A virus may damage the pancreas by directly attacking it. Indeed, there have been small outbreaks of type 1 diabetes that give support to this idea.

- ✔ As a result of normal chemical reactions in our bodies we produce highly reactive molecules called *oxygen free radicals*. Despite the name, we can assure you that they bear no similarity to hippies from 1960s Berkeley, California. Oxygen free radicals can be produced in excess numbers by exposure to air pollution and smoking.

> They can also be produced by exposure to high glucose levels and substances called *free fatty acids*. It is possible that oxygen free radicals accumulate in and damage the pancreas.
>
> ✔ Certain chemicals are known to cause type 1 diabetes. One such example is a rat poison called Vacor, which, if ingested, can damage the pancreas.

There are other theories as well, but the simple truth of the matter is that we don't know what has caused your type 1 diabetes. We do know, however, that there are certain underlying genetic characteristics that may make you more susceptible to getting type 1 diabetes. Individually they would not cause you to develop diabetes, but when taken together with some other trigger, they might. All of us have our genetic "blueprint" laid out for us in our DNA. And DNA in turn is made up of smaller portions called genes. It is our genes that cause us to be short or tall, blonde or brunette, blue- or brown-eyed, and so forth. People with type 1 diabetes are more likely to have certain types of genes called HLA-DR3 or HLA-DR4. Even though these sound like they should be pals with R2D2 and C3PO, they are not quite so foreign as that; indeed, 95 percent of people with type 1 diabetes have one of these genes.

The best possible illustration of how getting type 1 diabetes must be a combination of a genetic susceptibility *and* an environmental trigger is found in one extraordinarily simple fact. If you have type 1 diabetes and you have an identical twin (who would, therefore, have the same genes as you do), the likelihood of your twin getting type 1 diabetes is somewhere between 25 to 50 percent. If the cause was purely genetic, the odds would be 100 percent. Something else clearly must be at play here. But what? At this time, we simply do not know.

The great British prime minister, Benjamin Disraeli, may have been right when he said there are "lies, damn lies, and statistics," but when it comes to the inheritance of type 1 diabetes, certain statistics do seem to be true. In particular, if you have a parent or a (non-identical) sibling with type 1 diabetes you have approximately a 5-percent risk of developing type 1 diabetes. This risk rises to about 30 percent if *both* your parents have type 1 diabetes.

Preventing type 1 diabetes

It would give us untold pleasure to be able to make this the shortest chapter in this book. How wonderful to be able to write: "Take Vaccine X and you will be guaranteed to avoid type 1 diabetes." Well, we could write it but it would not be truthful. In fact there is no known way to prevent type 1 diabetes. But it is certainly not from lack of trying.

A variety of drugs (even including insulin) have been tried on people at high risk for developing type 1 diabetes, but these people ended up faring no better than those who did not receive the treatment.

Things are not all doom and gloom, however. Researchers are hard at work trying to solve the mystery of type 1 diabetes prevention. And unlike years ago, when scientists often worked in relative isolation, researchers now routinely pool their resources to improve their odds of success. Indeed, a new organization has been formed, TrialNet (www.diabetestrialnet.org) — of which the Hospital for Sick Children in Toronto is a member — that is "solely dedicated to testing new approaches to understanding, preventing and treating type 1 diabetes." This type of intensive, integrated approach by researchers is wonderful news, indeed.

You Have Type 2 Diabetes

Type 2 diabetes is much, much more common than type 1 diabetes (10 times more common, in fact). Whereas type 1 diabetes tends to develop in children and young adults, type 2 diabetes typically affects middle-aged or older people. Over the past 10 years, however, there has been an epidemic of type 2 diabetes in children and, remarkably, up to 25 percent (or, in some communities, even more) of kids with newly diagnosed diabetes have the type 2 variety. The reason why this is particularly sad is that type 2 diabetes is often avoidable and these children (some under the age of 10) might have been spared if they had played more hockey and basketball and spent less time watching television. If you have type 2 diabetes and want to help protect your young child or grandchild from also getting type 2 diabetes, perhaps for next year's birthday gift consider giving a YMCA/YWCA membership rather than a video game. Even better, while you're at it, get a membership for yourself, too, and go together!

When Paul, Anne's 10-year-old son, fell off the honour roll for the first time in four years, she thought it was time for him to start to buckle down on his homework. Anne spent extra time reviewing Paul's homework with him, but found it increasingly difficult to get her son to stay focused on his work. He seemed kind of fatigued, but otherwise healthy apart from his being considerably overweight. Anne herself had a weight problem and could readily relate to how tired it sometimes made her to carry her extra bulk around. As the semester went on, both Paul's marks and his energy continued going rapidly south, so Anne decided it was time to take her son to see a doctor. It took the doctor little time to find out what was wrong. "Anne, your son has diabetes; that's why he's not feeling right." Anne remembers how stunned she felt upon hearing the news. Diabetes? How could that be? That's what older people or underweight kids got, she thought. It was a shock to her to find out that overweight children are also prone to diabetes. Fortunately, both Anne and Paul were receptive to the types of changes they had to make to improve their health and they both immediately set about to lose weight and to exercise. What a thrill it was for them when within weeks they both felt newly energized and Paul was once again getting As.

With the type 2 diabetes condition, the pancreas is able to make insulin but the body's tissues are not able to use it properly. This is called _insulin resistance_, and we look at this in more detail later in this chapter.

It is crucial to know that if you have type 2 diabetes, you do not have a less severe or less important form of diabetes than if you had type 1 diabetes. You do not have a "touch of diabetes"; you have the real thing, meaning you require intensive therapy and equally intensive monitoring to keep you healthy. Don't let anyone try to convince you that if you are being treated with nutrition ("diet") therapy alone, your diabetes is less serious than if you were on insulin. On the other hand, do not let anyone try to convince you that if you are on insulin, your condition "must be worse" than someone with diabetes who does not require insulin. All diabetes is serious. All people with diabetes are at risk of complications, but, equally important, working with their health care team, they have the means to reduce that risk

Type 2 diabetes is written as, well, type 2 diabetes, not type II diabetes. The little in-joke amongst diabetes specialists is that this nomenclature was chosen so that doctors wouldn't think it was to be called type eleven diabetes!

Identifying the symptoms of type 2 diabetes

Nicholas had always been a very healthy man. Indeed, the last time he had seen a doctor was when he had his appendix taken out 10 years ago, when he was 40 years of age. The only reason he was now in the family doctor's office was at his wife's insistence. Starting a year ago, he had noticed some mild numbness in his right big toe. A month or two later, the same thing developed in his left big toe. Nicholas was not a complainer and he figured it was just because of some new, overly tight-fitting shoes he had yet to break in. Nonetheless, as the months passed, things got worse and worse and now the numbness involved all his toes and had started to feel increasingly painful. When his doctor examined Nicholas's feet they looked healthy enough, but when the doctor pressed on the toes with a thin nylon rod, Nicholas hardly noticed. A few tests later and the doctor had made her diagnosis. Nicholas had diabetes. It was a shock for Nicholas. He had no recollection of having been overly thirsty or passing excessive quantities of urine. Indeed, he had felt perfectly fine otherwise. Not in a million years had he imagined that diabetes could show itself in such an unusual way.

Unlike type 1 diabetes, the symptoms of type 2 diabetes tend to come on gradually; often so gradually that people who later discover they have the condition have discounted the symptoms, blaming them on something else. Perhaps before you were diagnosed as having type 2 diabetes, you attributed your weight loss to a new diet you had put yourself on. Or maybe you remember blaming your thirst on a particularly hot summer. Indeed, the symptoms of type 2 diabetes can come on so gradually and so imperceptibly that by the time it is discovered, your blood glucose may be extraordinarily high and, moreover, may have been high for so long that damage has already occurred to your body. In fact, up to 50 percent of people newly diagnosed with type 2 diabetes *already* have some degree of damage to their bodies. (It is for this reason that the Canadian Diabetes Association recommends people be routinely screened for diabetes; the goal is to try to make the diagnosis as early as possible so that treatment can be given before damage to the body occurs.)

Many of the symptoms of (uncontrolled) type 2 diabetes are common to type 1 diabetes, including the following:

- Frequent urination
- Increase in thirst
- Weight loss and increased hunger
- Fatigue
- Blurred vision

Weight loss is more common with newly diagnosed type 1 diabetes but also occurs fairly frequently with type 2 diabetes. There are some other differences in symptoms, and the following ones are much more likely to be present with type 2 diabetes:

- **Slow wound healing**: If you have high blood glucose levels, your body's ability to heal itself becomes impaired and you may find that seemingly minor cuts don't heal as quickly as they used to.

- **Yeast infections of the vagina and penis:** High glucose levels make the genital areas of your body prone to yeast infections. In a woman this may manifest as a vaginal discharge and, in a man, as a reddish rash at the end of the penis (balanitis).

- **Numbness of the feet:** This is not so much a symptom of high blood glucose as it is a symptom of nerve damage. If you have had high blood glucose levels for a number of years you may develop an uncomfortable burning or numb feeling in your feet. As Nicholas (in the preceding anecdote) discovered, this can be the first clue alerting you to the fact that you not only have diabetes, but that it has been there for quite some time.

Investigating the causes of type 2 diabetes

Although finding the initial trigger leading to type 1 diabetes has proved very elusive, we know a lot more about why people develop type 2 diabetes.

When you were told you had diabetes you may have thought of relatives of yours who shared the same problem. Indeed, you may have thought of *many* relatives who had diabetes. What you and your extended family have in common is, of course, more than being at risk for diabetes. You share many *genes* in common, including those that make you prone to getting diabetes. Note that the fact that your father or mother or sister or brother may have diabetes does *not* guarantee that you, too, will get it, but it does increase your risk.

If you have a parent with type 2 diabetes you have approximately a 15-percent risk of developing type 2 diabetes. This risk rises to about 50 percent if *both* your parents have type 2 diabetes. If you have a sibling with type 2 diabetes your risk is only 10 percent, but — and this is startling — if your sibling is your identical twin, your risk of developing type 2 diabetes rises to 90 percent. But before you throw your hands up in despair, please note there is a very, very large "but" here.

The "but" is that there is more to getting type 2 diabetes than family background alone. In addition to having relatives with diabetes, most people who acquire type 2 diabetes are overweight and sedentary. And we have recent scientific studies showing overwhelming evidence that your risk of developing type 2 diabetes can be drastically reduced by making appropriate lifestyle changes. Just like Tom Cruise discovers in the movie *Minority Report*, we have control over our destiny. (We discuss this further in the next section, on prevention.)

In the early stages of type 2 diabetes your pancreas produces large quantities of insulin. The main problem is that the insulin is not working effectively. Insulin is like a key that opens up the cells (especially your fat and muscle cells) to allow glucose to enter. In type 2 diabetes this key is malfunctioning. This is called insulin resistance (see "You Have the Metabolic Syndrome" below for a further discussion on this topic).

Thrifty genes

In countries where people do not get enough food, people whose genetic makeup enables their bodies to use carbohydrates in a very efficient manner have an advantage over the rest of the population because they can survive on the low food and calorie supplies. When these people finally receive ample supplies of food, their bodies are overwhelmed and they are more likely to become fat and develop diabetes. This may explain why people in developing countries are the most at risk to develop type 2 diabetes. The same theory may explain why First Nations have a higher risk of developing diabetes. This proposal is called the *thrifty gene hypothesis.*

Although the initial problem with type 2 diabetes is that your insulin is not working properly, as time passes the pancreas also runs into difficulties and eventually cannot make enough insulin. That is one of the main reasons that so many people with type 2 diabetes end up requiring insulin as time goes by. If you have type 2 diabetes and you require insulin to keep your blood glucose levels under control, this does **not** mean you have failed. It is not your fault. It simply means that your pancreas is unable to produce sufficient insulin for your body's needs.

People often think that sugar and stress cause type 2 diabetes, but in fact, they don't. Eating excessive amounts of sugar may bring out the disease to the extent that it makes you overweight, but that is quite different from saying sugar "causes diabetes." Indeed, eating too much protein or fat will do the same thing. As for excess stress, it can make your glucose control worse *if* you already have diabetes, but it does not *cause* diabetes.

Preventing type 2 diabetes

Unlike type 1 diabetes, type 2 diabetes can be prevented, or at the very least delayed, according to recent medical studies.

Type 2 diabetes almost always occurs in people who are overweight and sedentary. Like anything in life, there are exceptions, but over 90 percent of the time this is the case. However, by losing weight and exercising regularly you can reduce your risk of developing type 2 diabetes by over 50 per-cent. If you already have type 2 diabetes, then do your loved ones a favour and share this information with them so they can start to consider making the necessary lifestyle changes to help them avoid getting (or at least delaying the onset of) type 2 diabetes.

To achieve this huge reduction in risk, all you need to do is lose 5 percent of your body weight and exercise for 150 min-utes per week (which is only about 21 minutes a day)!

Research reveals that prevention is most likely to succeed with lifestyle therapy (that is; weight loss and exercise), but we must say that this is often the most difficult prescription of all. Fortunately, these same studies show that you can still achieve nearly similar benefit by using certain medications (such as metformin, or acarbose).

The medical studies just alluded to looked at people who already had problems with elevated blood glucose levels. They had *pre-diabetes*, meaning their readings were higher than normal but not high enough to classify them as having diabetes. We talk more about this condition later in this chapter.

There are several ways to determine whether or not you are overweight including:

- **Body Mass Index (BMI):** This is the most commonly used technique to determine if someone is overweight. Basically, BMI is an indicator of whether you are the right weight for your height. It can be calculated — though nobody ever does it this way — by dividing your weight in kilograms by the square of your height in metres. Uh-huh. Realistically, you can just look it up on a graph (see Figure 3-1) or use an online calculator (www.nhlbisupport.com/bmi/bminojs.htm). A normal BMI is 18.5 to 24.9. Note that the normal range for BMI does NOT apply to pregnant or breastfeeding woman, nor does it apply to infants, children, or adolescents (nor to particularly muscular individuals).

- **Waist circumference:** Another way to establish whether you are overweight is to measure your waist circumfer-ence. Your health risk goes up if your waist circumference is equal to or greater than 88 centimetres (35 inches) for women, 102 centimetres (40 inches) for men.

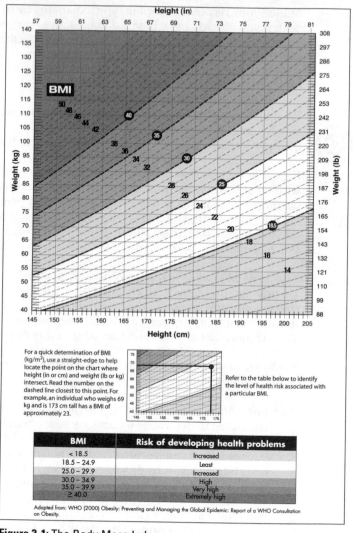

Figure 3-1: The Body Mass Index.

When it comes to having too much fat in your body, not all fat is equal. If you have extra fat around your belly but not over other areas of your body, that puts you at much higher risk of getting type 2 diabetes than if you had extra weight distributed over all parts of your body. This is because fat over your mid-section is more likely to cause insulin resistance (which we discuss in the preceding section and will discuss further later in this chapter).

Knowledge is power. And now that you know the main risk factors leading to type 2 diabetes, you have the ability to lessen the likelihood of getting it. And if you already have it, reducing your BMI and your extra fat tissue can markedly improve your health anyhow. The point of finding out your BMI is not that you should get angry or frustrated with yourself. Rather, you know what the problem is and can now take steps (both figurative and literal) to improve it.

Key Differences Between Type 1 and Type 2 Diabetes

There are many similarities between type 1 and type 2 diabetes; however, there are also some important differences. The following table highlights some of these differences. (Please note there are *many* exceptions to these):

Table 3-1	Differences Between Type 1 and Type 2 Diabetes	
	Type 1 diabetes	*Type 2 diabetes*
Age at time of diagnosis	Less than 20	More than 40
Length of time present before diagnosis	Months	Years
Weight status at time of diagnosis	Normal or underweight	Overweight
Most common symptoms at time of diagnosis	Thirst, frequent urination, weight loss	Thirst, frequent urination, visual blurring
Insulin defect	Insufficient insulin ("beta cell failure")	Ineffective insulin ("insulin resistance")
Antibodies present to insulin and/or islet cells	Yes	No
Family history of diabetes	Sometimes	Almost always
Initial therapy	Lifestyle & insulin	Lifestyle (with or without medication)

You Have the Metabolic Syndrome

Over the past several years a number of pieces of a puzzle have been found to fit together. Researchers have observed that people who have insulin resistance are prone to developing not only type 2 diabetes but other health problems as well (including conditions as varied as heart disease and infertility). This problem is called the Metabolic Syndrome.

In your Internet travels you may have come across other names for this condition. One is "Insulin Resistance Syndrome." This term has not yet come into common use. Another name is "Syndrome X." The problem with this term is that there is more than one type of health condition called Syndrome X. You'd think there was a shortage of letters in the alphabet! Anyhow, to avoid confusion, it is best to refer to the metabolic syndrome as, well, the metabolic syndrome.

The definition of the Metabolic Syndrome is in evolution (that is a nice way to say that doctors can't agree on it), but it is usually considered to be present if you have *three or more* of the following:

- ✔ Fasting blood glucose of 6.1 mmol/L or higher

- ✔ Blood pressure of 130/85 or higher

- ✔ Triglycerides of 1.7 mmol/L or higher (triglycerides are one of the fats in the blood)

- ✔ HDL cholesterol (the "good" type of cholesterol) less than 1.0 mmol/L (for men) or less than 1.3 mmol/L (for women)

- ✔ Abdominal obesity (as defined as a waist circumference of more than 102 cm — about 40 inches — for men; more than 88 cm — about 35 inches — for women)

If you have the Metabolic Syndrome, take that to be a wake-up call: You need to make crucial lifestyle interventions to reduce your risk of the condition deteriorating into diabetes, heart attacks, and other serious health issues. Your destiny is largely in your hands (and brain, in a manner of speaking). We talk more about the various ways to improve your health throughout this book. In particular, we address weight issues in Chapter 7.

You Have Pre-diabetes

You may be tolerant of your children and you may be tolerant of your neighbours and workmates. Heck, you may be the most tolerant person in the world but, alas, that does not mean you are tolerant of your glucose. With impaired glucose tolerance (IGT), you could say, to paraphrase Hamlet, "Diabetes or not diabetes; that is the question." If you have IGT, your post-meal blood glucose levels are not high enough to say you have diabetes, but not low enough to be normal either. In other words, when you have IGT, your diabetes (or not diabetes) future is being decided.

A physician will diagnose IGT if you have a blood glucose of 7.8 to 11.0 mmol/L two hours after drinking 75 grams of glucose. A related condition (with similar implications and importance) is *impaired fasting glucose* (IFG) which is diagnosed if your blood glucose is 6.1 to 6.9 after not having ingested any calories for the preceding eight hours. *Pre-diabetes* is a very recently coined term and refers to both impaired fasting glucose and impaired glucose tolerance.

Pre-diabetes is important to know about for two main reasons:

✔ **High risk of developing type 2 diabetes:** Think of pre-diabetes as an early warning system. It is an alert that you are at high risk of getting type 2 diabetes. Indeed, the risk of pre-diabetes developing into type 2 diabetes is as much as 10 percent in any year and about 90 percent over 10 years (hence the reason for calling this condition "pre-diabetes"). Not good odds, eh? But there is a "but": despite the name, pre-diabetes does *not* have to progress to type 2 diabetes. As you read in the preceding section, appropriate lifestyle (and sometimes, medication) intervention can halt (or, at the very least, slow down) this progression.

✔ **High risking of developing damaged blood vessels:** Having pre-diabetes puts you at very high risk of developing hardening of the arteries (atherosclerosis), which can ultimately lead to heart attacks, strokes, and amputations. However, this does *not* have to happen. Aggressive treatment of pre-diabetes and other risk factors for vascular disease can keep you healthy. This means paying attention to your diet, being physically active, making sure your blood pressure and lipids (cholesterol and triglycerides) are good, and, of course, not smoking.

Although the term "pre-diabetes" is very apt in that it hammers home the message that IFG and IGT are huge risk factors for getting type 2 diabetes, it implies an inevitability about something that we know is not necessarily inevitable. IFG and IGT do *not* have to lead to diabetes.

Chapter 4

Dealing with Acute Glucose Problems

••

In This Chapter

▶ Knowing when problems with glucose control become an emergency

▶ Dealing with low blood glucose

••

Glucose control in diabetes involves two separate issues. On the one hand, there is your long-term goal of maintaining good glucose levels to feel well and to avoid damaging the body as time goes by. On the other hand, there are those situations when glucose control suddenly deteriorates and requires urgent attention. In this chapter we discuss those circumstances that require immediate action.

Hypoglycemia (Low Blood Glucose)

Hypoglycemia is an oft-misunderstood term that gets thrown about with the randomness of a knuckle-ball pitch on a windy day. (You may notice as you read this book that references to hockey keep appearing. But, lest we offend fans of the Toronto Blue Jays, we thought we'd throw in this baseball analogy.) Many people mistakenly believe that hypoglycemia leads to diabetes. So let's set the record straight. It doesn't. Remember, you read it here first.

Hypoglycemia is defined as a blood glucose level below normal. That much is straight-forward. The problem is defining precisely how low a normal blood glucose can be. This is a subject of some controversy in the medical community, with numbers ranging from 2.5 to 4.0 mmol/L having been proposed, however the current guidelines issued by the Canadian Diabetes Association (www.diabetes.ca) consider hypglycemia to be a blood glucose level of 4.0 mmol/L or less.

Your body doesn't function well when you have too little glucose in your blood. Your brain needs glucose to allow you to think properly, and your muscles need the energy that glucose provides in much the same way that your car needs gasoline to run. So, when your body detects that it has low blood glucose, it sends out a group of hormones that fight to raise your glucose level. But if you're taking medication to reduce your blood glucose (see later in this chapter), those hormones have to fight the strength of the diabetes medication that has been pushing down your glucose levels.

Not every person develops symptoms of hypoglycemia at the same level of blood glucose. Some people notice it at blood glucose levels of 3.8, others only when their blood glucose level is between 2 and 3. Moreover, a person might notice it on one occasion when his or her blood glucose level is below 3.6 and that *same* person might not notice it on another occasion until it is below 3.2. It is crucial also to remember that glucose meters are not perfect. You may have already discovered that you can check your reading seconds apart and find discrepancies of up to 15 percent. That does not mean your blood glucose level changed that much in that brief interval. It simply means the machines are not precision instruments. (Your machine, how-ever, should not give readings — checked moments apart — that differ by *more than* 15 percent. If it does, have your device checked to make sure it is not malfunctioning.)

Symptoms of hypoglycemia

Doctors traditionally divide the symptoms of hypoglycemia into two major categories:

> ✔ **Symptoms that are due to the effects of the hormones (especially epinephrine, also called adrenaline) that your body sends out to counter the glucose-lowering effect of insulin.** These are called *autonomic* symptoms.

> ✓ **Symptoms that are due to your brain not receiving enough fuel with the result that your intellectual function suffers**. These are called *neuroglycopenic symptoms,* derived from *neuro* (referring to the nervous system), *glyco* (glucose), and *penic* (insufficient).

Autonomic symptoms are your best friends. They are your warning system alerting you to a problem of low blood glucose and demanding you attend to it, before it progresses to the more dangerous neuroglycopenic stage (which we discuss shortly).

Autonomic symptoms are:

- ✓ Trembling (shaking of your body; especially of the hands)
- ✓ Palpitations (noticing a rapid or excessively forceful heartbeat)
- ✓ Sweating
- ✓ Anxiety
- ✓ Hunger
- ✓ Nausea
- ✓ Tingling

As you look through the above list, you may recognize having had some or all of these symptoms at various times in your life, even if you have never been on medicine that could cause low blood glucose. The reason: these symptoms can occur in *any* circumstance where epinephrine levels are high, and that includes so-called "fight or flight" situations where you are under extreme stress. (Examples are if you are about to write a difficult exam, about to have a job interview, or, let's say you were Ed Belfour and you look up and see Jarome Iginla coming toward you on a breakaway . . .)

Shortly after you begin therapy for high blood glucose you may find that you are experiencing autonomic symptoms, suggesting you have hypoglycemia even though your blood glucose levels may not be low. This is perfectly normal — it will take a few days for your body to become accustomed to having normal blood glucose levels, at which point your symptoms will resolve.

Neuroglycopenic symptoms are much more of a problem. These symptoms are most definitely not your friends. Quite the opposite. Whereas autonomic symptoms alert you to a problem, neuroglycopenic symptoms often interfere with your ability to recognize and deal with hypoglycemia. By the time these symptoms develop, your blood glucose level is usually profoundly low and has become a true emergency. These symptoms include:

- Difficulty concentrating
- Confusion
- Weakness
- Drowsiness
- Vision changes (such as double vision or loss of vision)
- Difficulty speaking
- Headache
- Dizziness
- Tiredness

People lose their ability to think clearly when they become hypoglycemic. They make simple errors, and other people often assume that they are drunk. Suffice to say, if Albert Einstein were having an episode of hypoglycemia, he may have ended up mistakenly deciding E = mc or, in keeping with our hockey analogy, Wayne Gretzky would have been the not-quite-as-Great One. Fortunately, adult brains have an amazing capacity to put up with insults like hypoglycemia, and long-term damage to the brain from low blood glucose almost never occurs. Because the brains of infants and young children are more sensitive to injury, however, it is especially important to avoid severe hypoglycemia in this age group (see the following list for a definition of severe hypoglycemia).

Hypoglycemia can be classified as:

- **Mild:** Autonomic symptoms are present and you are able to treat yourself.

- **Moderate:** Autonomic and neuroglycopenic symptoms are present and you are able to treat yourself.

> ✔ **Severe:** Hypoglycemia is bad enough that you require someone else to assist you. Unconsciousness may occur. (With severe hypoglycemia the blood glucose is typically less than 2.8 mmol/L.)

One of Alan's patients was driving on a highway when another driver noticed that she was weaving back and forth in her lane and reported her to the highway patrol. A patrolman stopped her, concluded that she was drunk, and took her to jail. Fortunately, someone noticed that she was wearing a diabetes medical alert bracelet. After promptly receiving the glucose that she needed, she rapidly recovered. No charges were filed, but clearly this is a situation that you want to avoid.

If you take medicines that can cause hypoglycemia, for your own safety it would be very wise to wear a medical alert bracelet or necklace. At the very least (and it is certainly not as good), carry some form of identification in your purse or wallet noting that you have diabetes. You may never need them, but it is a good idea to be prepared just in case.

Most people with diabetes go their entire lives without ever experiencing even a single episode of *severe* hypoglycemia. The vast majority of the time if hypoglycemia is being experienced the early-warning, autonomic symptoms kick in and allow you to quickly rectify the problem.

If you are on medications such as insulin or glyburide (glyburide is a type of oral hypoglycemic agent), it is quite possible that you recall having had at least one episode where your hands started to shake, you became sweaty and hungry, and you recognized that something wasn't quite right. You probably reached for your glucose meter, checked your blood glucose level, and found it be somewhere in the low 3's. You likely took some sugar candies or a glass of juice or pop and felt better within a few minutes. Congratulations: you successfully diagnosed, treated, and cured your first patient. Feel free to write the rest of this chapter. Oh, never mind, we'll do it.

As we discuss earlier in this chapter, symptoms such as sweating or palpitations, which can indicate hypoglycemia, can also occur in situations, such as stress, where your blood glucose level may actually be perfectly normal. For that reason, it is very important to conclude that you have hypoglycemia only if you have demonstrated a low blood glucose level on your glucose meter.

Causes of hypoglycemia

Hypoglycemia does not cause diabetes. Now, in another attempt to dispel popular misconceptions, we wish to hereby announce that diabetes does not cause hypoglycemia. Remember, you read it here first. Certain medicines used to *treat* diabetes can cause hypoglycemia, but it is not caused by diabetes in and of itself. Indeed, if you have diabetes and are being treated purely with lifestyle measures (nutrition and exercise therapy) you will *never* experience hypoglycemia.

Hypoglycemia is always unintended. Ideally, your blood glucose levels would always be normal — never high, never low. Unfortunately, we seldom have that degree of success with our imperfect therapies. Most of the medicines we use to prevent blood glucose levels from being too high have the potential to drop them too low. This is especially likely if you are taking any of the following:

- **Sulfonylurea medicine:** Medicines from this family (the most commonly prescribed of which is a drug called *glyburide*) have the potential to cause low blood glucose.

- **Insulin:** Unlike insulin made by your pancreas, insulin you inject does not have the ability to turn itself off the instant you no longer need it. An injection of insulin will help to reduce your blood glucose level, but it also has the potential to drop your level excessively. This is called an "insulin reaction." You may have heard the term "insulin shock" used in reference to particularly bad insulin reactions. Insulin shock is not a scientific term, however, and can be misleading. Accordingly, we will not be using it beyond this brief explanation.

- **Meglitinides & D-phenylalanine derivatives:** Never do we, as diabetes specialists, consider ourselves luckier than when we attend conferences where these medicines are discussed. Oh no, not just because they are important drugs to know about. No. We consider ourselves fortunate because it is at these conferences that we learn how to pronounce them! Don't worry; no one uses these names anyhow. Doctors pretty well just use the trade names (Gluconorm, Starlix) for drugs currently available within this group. These drugs, like sulfonylureas, make the pancreas release extra insulin and have the potential to cause hypoglycemia.

Non-diabetes causes of hypoglycemia

Hypoglycemia can occur for many other reasons quite unrelated to diabetes treatment. Fasting hypoglycemia can, for example, occur with certain types of tumours.

Hypoglycemia developing a few hours after eating is called reactive hypoglycemia and is generally treated by eating more frequent, smaller meals.

Other commonly used drugs such as metformin (Glucophage) or thiazolidinediones (another impossibly difficult name to pronounce; just call them TZD's and doctors will know what you are referring to) do not cause hypoglycemia unless they are being used in combination with medicines from the list above.

There are many unfair things about having diabetes. It is unfair to get it. It is unfair to develop complications. And it is especially unfair that those people with diabetes who try the hardest to stay healthy are the most prone to getting hypoglycemia. If you have poorly controlled glucose levels with values running between 15 and 20, you may not feel great, but you are highly, highly unlikely ever to run into significant problems with hypoglycemia. But if you look after yourself meticulously and are keeping your blood glucose levels in the 4 to 8 range, you are at much greater risk of having hypoglycemia. Fortunately, it is possible to have excellent control and, at the same time, to minimize the risk of getting hypoglycemia. It ain't easy, but it is doable. We discuss this further later in this chapter.

Treatment of hypoglycemia

The vast majority of episodes of hypoglycemia are mild and you will be able to deal with them easily.

If you find that your blood glucose level is low, then it is imperative that you ingest some sugar to restore your level to normal. The Canadian Diabetes Association (CDA) recommends that if you have mild to moderate hypoglycemia (that is, you are still awake and aware enough to take things by mouth) you should take the following steps:

✔ **Step One:** Eat or drink 15 grams (10 grams for children less than 5 years of age or less than 20 kg; that is, less than 44 pounds) of a fast-acting carbohydrate such as:

- Three 5-gram glucose tablets (for example, BD glucose tablets)

- Five 3-gram glucose tablets (for example, Dextrosol tablets)

- 175 mL (3⁄4 cup) of juice or regular (not diet or sugar-free) pop (but, see the tip below)

- 15 mL (3 tsp) honey

- 15 mL (3 tsp) table sugar dissolved in water

✔ **Step Two:** Wait 10 to 15 minutes, and then retest your blood. If your blood glucose level is still less than 4 mmol/L, ingest another 15 grams (10 grams for small children) of carbohydrate.

✔ **Step Three:** If your next meal is more than 1 hour away, or you are going to be physically active, eat a snack, such as half a sandwich or cheese and crackers. The snack should contain 15 grams of carbohydrate and a source of protein.

Despite what most people think (and do), orange juice is not as effective as products like Dextrosol because it is slower to raise glucose levels and relieve you of symptoms. Nonetheless, if you have some O.J. and it's handier than an alternative, it will work.

If you are being treated with acarbose (Prandase) and you develop hypoglycemia you should be treated with glucose (such as Dextrosol), not sucrose (such as fruit juice).

If you are hypoglycemic and you're about to eat a meal, you should *still* treat your hypoglycemia with fast-acting carbohydrate as described above. This will ensure that your blood glucose is brought up rapidly.

Because the symptoms of hypoglycemia are so unpleasant and because hypoglycemia is understandably scary, you may find yourself taking candy after candy until you feel better without actually giving time for the first "treatment" to take effect. Then, when all that sugar you have just ingested gets absorbed into your system, you may find that your glucose level is up into the teens. It is best, therefore, to give the first treatment a few minutes to work before you take another.

Because your mental state may be impaired when you have hypoglycemia, you need to make sure that your friends or relatives know in advance what hypoglycemia is and what to do about it. This is especially important if your hypoglycemia is so severe that you are unconscious or nearly so, in which case you will be unable to swallow properly. In this circumstance, people should *not* try to feed you, because you could choke. Instead, your helper should administer glucagon (see below) to you and/or call 9-1-1 to summon an ambulance. If you experience milder hypoglycemia, where you are alert but somewhat confused and unable to obtain an appropriate sugar source, then your helper simply needs to find one for you and help you to ingest it.

Inform people about your diabetes and about how to recognize hypoglycemia. Let them know where you store your emergency supplies (such as the glucose tablets you use to treat hypoglycemia). Don't keep your diabetes a secret. The people close to you will be glad to know how to help you.

Glucagon is available by prescription from pharmacies in a package called a glucagon kit. This kit includes a syringe and 1 mg of glucagon, one of the major hormones that raises glucose, which your helper should inject into your leg muscle. (Half that dose – that is, 0.5 mg – should be used if you are treating a child five years of age or less.) The injection of glucagon raises the blood glucose and within 15–20 minutes you will likely become fully alert. Be sure to check the expiry date marked on the glucagon kit to make certain that it hasn't become outdated if you haven't used it for a long time.

If you have just experienced a severe episode of hypoglycemia and you required an injection of glucagon, then once you have fully come around and are again able to swallow properly, you should consume some quick-acting hypoglycemia treatment (see the list earlier in this section) followed by food to help prevent your redeveloping hypoglycemia as the glucagon wears off.

Some people are, understandably, just too nervous or too intimidated to take it upon themselves to administer glucagon. In that case, they should just call an ambulance.

Remember that when you pick up the glucagon kit from the pharmacy, the person that is most likely to be giving it should go with you. The pharmacist MUST sit down and explain to both of you how it is to be given.

If you live, work, or play in an area where emergency health care services are more than just minutes away, it is especially important for you to have a glucagon kit. Do you snowmobile? Hunt? Hike? Boat? Do you live in a remote area? Does your job take you into the bush? All of these situations would warrant having a supply of glucagon readily available. Keep in mind the Boy Scouts' motto: "Be prepared."

If you have experienced severe hypoglycemia — even if you quickly recovered — it is crucial that you notify your family physician or your diabetes specialist so that they can make appropriate adjustments to your therapy to lessen the likelihood of your having another severe attack. If you are feeling well and have fully recovered from the episode, you do not have to call your health care team right away, but it would be wise to get in touch with them within a day or two.

Preventing hypoglycemia

Not everyone with diabetes experiences hypoglycemia. As we discussed earlier in this chapter, if you are being treated with lifestyle therapy alone, you will not have low blood glucose. However, most people with diabetes at some point will require use of medicines (such as insulin or glyburide) that will put them at risk of hypoglycemia. Although there is no foolproof way to avoid hypoglycemia, there are a few techniques to remember:

✔ **Do not miss or delay meals:** Because pills and insulin that are used to reduce blood glucose do not have the good sense to know exactly when to stop working, like the famous battery-operated bunny they sometimes tend to keep going and going. (Precisely how long depends on the particular type of pill or insulin that you are using.) That would be fine if your glucose level is still high, but not so fine if your level has come back to normal, as it most likely will have by the time your next meal rolls around. If your meal is unduly delayed, the medicine may pull your glucose level down too low.

✔ **Have a bedtime snack:** Eating a bedtime snack is not necessary for most people with diabetes unless you are taking evening doses of insulin and your bedtime blood glucose level is less than 7 mmol/L in which case a bedtime snack containing at least 15 grams of carbohydrate and 15 grams of protein will help you avoid having a low reading overnight. If you find that going to bed with a higher glucose level does not prevent overnight lows then you should take a snack even if your bedtime reading is higher than 7 mmol/L. (If you are on insulin it is a good idea to periodically test your blood glucose level at about 3 a.m. to make sure it is not going low overnight without your having recognized it.)

✔ **Plan your exercise:** Exercise is an essential component of your diabetes therapy (particularly if you have type 2 diabetes), but it is important for you to be aware that exercise accelerates the rate at which glucose moves from the blood into muscle (where it is used as fuel) and, thus, can cause you to have hypoglycemia. By all means *do* exercise; however, if you know from experience that when you perform a certain type or amount of exercise you develop hypoglycemia, speak to your diabetes educator or physician about how to adjust your medicines or diet to reduce the risk of developing low blood glucose. Often the solution is something as simple as having a small snack before you work out. The worst thing is to have hypoglycemia every time you exercise; we can't imagine a stronger disincentive to exercising than that!

✔ **Avoid (or minimize) the use of other drugs that can cause hypoglycemia:** There are several drugs (not specifically being used to treat your diabetes) that you may take from time to time that have the potential to lower your blood glucose levels. These drugs include alcohol and *high* doses of aspirin (ASA). We discuss alcohol further in Chapter 7. If you are experiencing hypoglycemia, make sure you review *all* your medicines (and any alternative and complementary therapies) with your doctor to see if some changes should be made.

If you are on intensified insulin therapy, episodes of hypoglycemia are inevitable. Ian has found that, as a very rough rule of thumb, to achieve excellent overall blood glucose control you can expect to have *mild* hypoglycemia about two times per week. More frequent hypoglycemia may put you at undue risk of severe hypoglycemia. On the other hand, if you are on intensified insulin therapy and you are *never* experiencing episodes of hypoglycemia, your average blood glucose level is probably too high.

Hypoglycemia unawareness

Samantha was a 28-year-old patient of Ian's. She had developed diabetes when she was only 5 years of age. Samantha was a highly motivated patient and was monitoring her blood glucose levels many times per day. With aggressive use of insulin, nutrition therapy, and exercise she was able to keep her glucose readings between 3.8 and 6.6. Recently, while she was at work, her boss had found her staring vacantly into space. He was able to get her to drink some juice and she quickly came around, but the next day the same thing happened again. Two days later, her husband awakened to find Samantha soaking wet in bed beside him. He couldn't awaken her. He tested her blood and found her glucose level to be 1.8. He gave her an injection of glucagon (see above for a discussion about glucagon) and over the next 15 minutes she gradually awakened. Later that day, she went to see Ian in the office, her therapy was adjusted, and soon thereafter she was able to once again recognize when her blood glucose levels were too low.

Samantha's story is quite typical of patients with *hypoglycemia unawareness*. As the name suggests, this is a condition where you lose your ability to recognize when your blood glucose level has fallen below normal. This can occur for several reasons:

✔ **Repeated hypoglycemia:** If you have been experiencing frequent hypoglycemia — even if mild — your autonomic warning system (such as sweating and palpitations; see above) may start to fail and the first clue that you have low blood glucose can be when you are confused and unable to look after yourself.

✔ **Longstanding diabetes:** Occasionally, if you have had diabetes for a very long time (generally speaking, we are talking decades), your autonomic warning system may fail and, as in the situation above, the first clue there is a problem may be when you become confused.

✔ **Other drugs impairing your ability to recognize hypoglycemia:** Several drugs can interfere with your body's ability to produce autonomic symptoms. Such drugs include beta blockers (such as Inderal), which are often used to treat heart disease and high blood pressure. Another drug that some of you may have passing acquaintance with is alcohol, which, if used in sufficient quantities to impair your alertness, can blunt your ability to recognize when you are hypoglycemic.

Fortunately, in *almost* all cases you can restore your ability to recognize hypoglycemia. Sometimes it is simply a matter of avoiding alcohol. Other times it is adjusting your medicines.

Ketoacidosis

If you have type 1 diabetes, you are at risk for developing a temporary condition called *ketoacidosis*. Ketoacidosis (abbreviated DKA) is a condition in which your blood glucose level is high (typically above 14) *and* you have excess quantities of a type of acid called ketones in the blood. High blood glucose *without* the presence of ketones does not indicate DKA. (Though, of course it might indicate your glucose control is pretty crummy, but that is a different story.)

Ketoacidosis requires urgent attention because, if severe, it can be life threatening. Occasionally, the first clue that you have type 1 diabetes is when you become ill with ketoacidosis. More commonly DKA occurs after you already know that you have the disease.

The main source of energy for your muscles is glucose. And for glucose to be used properly you must have sufficient insulin in your body. If you have type 1 diabetes you lack the ability to produce insulin and, thus, you need to give it to yourself by injection.

But what happens if your body requires more insulin than you are giving? Several things can happen. Your blood glucose levels will climb (because the glucose cannot get into your cells without sufficient insulin to help it). Your body will start to break down fat (and muscle) because it cannot use glucose as a fuel. And, as fat tissue breaks down, it releases acids ("ketones") into the bloodstream. The result is that you develop ketoacidosis.

Symptoms of ketoacidosis

Depending on the severity of your DKA you will have some combination of the following symptoms:

- ✓ **Nausea, vomiting, and abdominal pain:** It is noteworthy that many people with diabetes — and many doctors also, by the way — mistakenly attribute these symptoms to "stomach flu" (*gastroenteritis*) even when it is due to DKA. (Of course you *may* simply have "the flu," but a doctor should come to this conclusion only after DKA has been discounted.)

- ✓ **Rapid breathing:** You experience rapid breathing when your blood is so acidic that your body tries to compensate by ridding itself of acids through the lungs.

- ✓ **Fruity breath:** The presence of ketones in your system gives your breath a fruity, not unpleasant odour. Most people with DKA do not notice it even though it might be apparent to bystanders.

- ✓ **Extreme tiredness and drowsiness**: If your DKA is mild, your tiredness may also be mild, but as your DKA worsens you will feel increasingly drowsy, and if your DKA becomes severe you can lose consciousness.

The Canadian Diabetes Association recommends that people with type 1 diabetes test for ketones:

✔ During periods of acute illness

✔ When pre-meal blood glucose readings are above 14 mmol/L

✔ When symptoms of DKA (see above) are present

Ketoacidosis occurs rarely in type 2 diabetes. Nonetheless, if you have type 2 diabetes and you develop typical symptoms of DKA, it would be a good idea to check for ketones.

Ketones can be tested in either the urine (with Ketostix test strips) or, preferably, in the blood (with use of the Precision Xtra ketone testing meter made by Abbott Diabetes Care; www.medisense.com).

If you notice that you have some symptoms of ketoacidosis and you test your blood ketone level and find it to be elevated (0.6 mmol/L or higher), you should contact your health care team. In most cases, the safest and best thing to do is to be seen at the closest emergency department. However, if you are fortunate enough to be working with a diabetes nurse educator who is both trained — and empowered — to deal with DKA and is immediately available, you can first contact him or her for detailed advice (unless you are feeling particularly unwell in which case you should simply proceed directly to hospital).

Causes of ketoacidosis

Ketoacidosis is caused by a *relative* lack of insulin. And no, this does not mean that it is caused by your first cousin Sally not having enough insulin. (Though perhaps she doesn't. We wouldn't know.) When we say *relative* lack of insulin, we mean that the amount of insulin in your body — no matter how much there is — is not enough for your body's needs. It follows, then, that DKA will develop in one of two general circumstances:

✔ **You are missing insulin doses:** If you have type 1 diabetes, your pancreas is unable to manufacture insulin, so you must give yourself insulin. Because most types of injected insulin don't last all that long in the body, if you miss doses your body quickly detects this and your metabolism will promptly suffer. The occasional missed dose will not likely harm you, but if you miss several consecutive doses, you will be at substantial risk for developing DKA.

✔ **You are not taking high enough doses of insulin:** It is quite possible that day to day you give yourself a fairly similar quantity of insulin and get along quite nicely, thank you very much. That is great. But if you are experiencing some additional stress (emotional or, more commonly, physical) on your body, you will likely require higher doses of insulin to meet your body's increased needs. Examples would be if you develop, say, pneumonia or a kidney infection.

If you have type 1 diabetes, you are dependent on insulin injections not only to preserve your health, but to preserve your life. Even if you are feeling rotten and are eating nothing, you CANNOT forgo taking your insulin. In fact, you may need to give yourself *more* insulin than usual. The sickest patients that diabetes specialists ever see are those people with diabetes who, unfortunately, either weren't given this advice or knew it but didn't follow it.

Treatment of ketoacidosis

Ketoacidosis is a serious condition that requires very careful treatment. If you have mild DKA, you will possibly be treated as an outpatient under the very, very close supervision of your diabetes educator (see the preceding section). The following will probably be part of your treatment:

✔ **Ensuring proper hydration:** Achieved by making sure you are drinking sufficient quantities of fluids.

✔ **Giving yourself frequent insulin injections:** You may be asked to give yourself injections of rapid-acting insulin as often as every 2 hours.

✔ **Testing blood:** You will need to check your blood glucose and blood ketone levels often.

If you have anything more than mild DKA, you should be treated in a hospital. The treatment will consist of the following:

✔ **Ensuring proper hydration and sodium balance:** Achieved by intravenous administration of sodium-rich fluids.

✔ **Restoring proper potassium and mineral balance:** This is achieved by intravenous or oral administration of potassium and, at times, calcium, phosphate, magnesium, and bicarbonate.

✔ **Administering insulin:** This is usually done intravenously.

✔ **Testing blood:** Oh yes, where would we be without blood testing? You will likely be poked and prodded quite a bit, but fortunately that can usually be done by inserting a small tube into a blood vessel that can, in a sense, be turned on and off at will (sort of like a tap), so you may not have to be jabbed afresh each time.

✔ **Looking for the cause:** If the reason for your having developed DKA is not apparent (like missing insulin doses, for example) you may require additional blood and urine tests, X-rays, and so on to try to determine what may have triggered the episode (pneumonia, for example).

Prevention of ketoacidosis

How truly wonderful it is that what was once both unavoidable (and fatal!) is now almost always avoidable. It does, however, take a fair bit of effort to accomplish this. The key measures to prevent DKA are:

✔ **Monitor, monitor, monitor:** Often the earliest signs of developing DKA are rising blood glucose readings. If you are testing your blood frequently you may well detect a problem before it gets out of hand.

✔ **Take your insulin:** Whatever you do, do not fall into the trap of figuring that if you are feeling unwell and not eating or drinking properly, you do not need insulin. Trust us; you *do* require insulin. Sometimes less than usual, sometimes the same as usual, and often, more than usual.

Beth was a 13-year-old girl who had had type 1 diabetes for three years. After visiting a friend at a cottage she came down with terrible diarrhea. She spent the better part of the day on the toilet, but with her mom's encouragement, she was able to drink lots of fluids. Beth usually required three injections of insulin per day and her total daily dose of insulin was generally about 20 units. When she became ill, her blood glucose level rose to 22 and her blood started to test positive for ketones. Beth contacted her diabetes educator, who advised her to test her blood glucose every 2 hours and told her to take extra rapid-acting insulin every 2 hours if her blood glucose level was elevated. Over the next 12 hours she ended up taking an *extra* 30 units. By the next day, Beth was feeling back to normal, her glucose levels were normal, she had no ketones in the blood, her insulin doses were back to usual, and she was out playing with her friends. Beth was thrilled. Her mom was thrilled. Her educator and her doctors were thrilled. Everyone was thrilled, in fact, except for Beth's friend, who felt terribly guilty when they found out their lake water was contaminated with giardiasis ("Beaver Fever"). Ah, but we'll leave that to another book.

Chapter 5

Meet Your Diabetes Team

- -

In This Chapter

▶ Presenting *you*, the star and centre attraction of your diabetes team

▶ Introducing your teammates

▶ Finding out how you all can form a winning team

- -

To the best of our knowledge, no hockey team has ever won a gold medal at the Olympics by sending only one player onto the ice. Nor do we know of any team that ever won gold without having a coach, a general manager, and a slew of fans rooting along the way. And if an Olympic hockey team ever played without a trainer and an equipment manager, it surely must have been way back before Don Cherry put on his first red-checkered sport jacket (with matching lime-green tie, of course!). Heck, it must have been before Howie Morenz notched his first hat trick.

Now it may not be easy to make it onto an Olympic hockey team, but *you* can be the star of *your own* team. Indeed, you should be the star of your own diabetes health care team, because for you to succeed with your diabetes, you must not only be the captain of the team, you must have all the other players working with you. There is nothing second rate about coming home from the Olympics with a silver or bronze, but when it comes to your health, we should always be after the top prize.

In this chapter we will look at the different players on your health care team, starting with the first, second, and third star of each and every game. That would be — you guessed it — you.

The only hockey player we can recall that came close to matching your selection as first, second, and third star of the game is Maurice "the Rocket" Richard who was awarded all three stars back in 1944 after scoring all five Habs' goals in a 5–1 Montreal Canadiens playoff victory. Clearly, you are in rarefied company.

You Are the Captain of the Team

You may not have wanted to be captain of the team; heck, you didn't want to be on a diabetes team to start with, but here you are, the star of the team, and as you might imagine, with stardom come certain responsibilities. Leadership, for example. This is where diabetes differs from almost any other illness. If you have appendicitis, it is not very likely that you will be the one to order the X-ray, deliver the anesthetic, hold the scalpel, and put in the stitches. No, your role would be relatively passive as the experts around you tend to your needs. Diabetes is not like that.

When you have diabetes, *you* have to take charge. *You,* after all, live with you. Day and night. Night and day, too, we suspect. *You* are the one that ultimately decides what you will eat, when you will exercise, when you will test your blood glucose levels, when you will take your medicines, and so forth. Other people can offer advice, other people can prompt or even cajole you, but in the end, the decisions are yours. And with your keen and ongoing involvement in your health care, you will be helping yourself to receive the best possible therapy to achieve and maintain good health. Like we said, you are the star.

It may seem rather daunting for you to have so much responsibility placed upon your shoulders. And there may be times when you simply want people to tell you to "do this" and "do that." But with time and support you will grow into your role and become comfortable with it.

Before we move on to a discussion about your teammates' functions, let's summarize what *your* responsibilities are as captain of your health care team. This list may seem intimidating, but you will be surprised at how quickly these responsibilities can all become part of your normal day-to-day existence:

✔ **Follow your lifestyle treatment plan:** This means knowing what foods you should eat, how much, and how often. What exercises you should do and how often you should do them. How much weight — if any — you should lose and the best strategy to achieve this. How much alcohol you can safely drink. If you smoke and want to quit, what cessation strategies are available to you.

✔ **Monitor your blood glucose:** You should become familiar with how to test your blood, how often you should test, what your target blood glucose levels are, and, importantly, what you should be doing to achieve these targets. You should also make sure that you have your A1C checked every 3 months *and* that you find out the result. (We discuss blood glucose and A1C testing in Chapter 6.)

✔ **Keep track of your blood pressure:** Anytime someone checks your blood pressure, ask what it is and write it down. Become familiar with what your target blood pressure is, and if your readings are too high, ask your doctor how he or she is going to help you reduce it.

✔ **Keep track of your lipid levels:** As with your blood pressure, anytime someone tests your lipid levels, you should write them down. Also, you should speak to your doctor to know what your target levels are, and if you are not within those targets, ask your doctor how he or she is going to help you meet those goals.

✔ **Schedule visits to each member of your health care team:** How often you see each member of the team will depend on many circumstances, including your state of health. Anytime you meet with your health care providers (be it your family doctor, diabetes specialist, diabetes educator or other member of your health care team), be sure to ask them when they want you to return. It is best to book the return appointment *before* you leave the office *and* write down the details on your calendar as soon as you get home (or, for the technologically savvy, in your PDA before you leave the office).

✔ **Know about your medicines:** Every time you see a physician or diabetes educator, be sure to bring all your medicines with you. At the very least, bring a list of your medicines, making note of your drugs' names, dosages, and how many times per day you are taking them. Telling your doctor that you are "on a small blue pill once a day" and a "red capsule twice a day" tells your physician more about the state of your colour vision than the nature of your drugs.

✔ **Ask questions:** For you to function as an effective captain of your health care team, you must know how you are performing. And you can't know this without your teammates giving you feedback. So, before you leave an appointment, make sure you have a good understanding of what your health care provider has concluded. Don't accept vague phrases like "your blood pressure is okay" or "your cholesterol isn't bad" or "your sugars are reasonable." As diabetes specialists we can tell you that these terms are meaningless. Meaning*ful* would be to hear that your blood pressure is 125/85, your LDL is 2.4, and your A1C is 7.4.

Dress for success

You might normally think that "power-dressing" is something that is done on Bay Street, not in your doctor's office. Well, you may be amazed at how much more "power" you can have in making sure you get the attention you need by dressing for the occasion. We're not talking business suits here; we're talking "easy access." On the day of a doctor's appointment, you would be well served to dress in such a way that you can easily expose your arm (for a blood pressure measurement) and your feet (for assessment of skin health, circulation, sensation, and so on. Even better, take off your shoes and socks while you are waiting for your doctor to come into the examining room; this will ensure that your feet will get looked at. (Of course, you will not want to do this if the doctor you are seeing is your eye doctor!) You may reasonably conclude that none of this dressing (and undressing) strategy should be necessary and we would agree completely. But in truth, if this technique makes it more likely your blood pressure or feet get checked, it may be a life- and limb-saving measure.

Your physician is dealing with many patients each day and even the most conscientious, well-meaning doctor can easily forget some of the specific issues that surround your particular situation. Therefore, be sure to bring up any concerns or questions you have about your health. Tell your doctor if you are having a problem such as chest pain, numbness in your feet, sexual dysfunction, and so forth. Otherwise, a potentially serious problem may end up being overlooked.

 When it comes to your health care, never accept the old adage that "no news is good news." Sometimes, no news means the lab lost your blood sample! If you have had tests done, follow up with your doctor (in person, by phone, by fax, by e-mail, or some other means) to obtain and discuss the results.

The remainder of this chapter looks at the responsibilities of the other members of your health care team. As you see what their roles are, you will further understand the ways that you can help *them* help *you*. After all, as the old expression says, knowledge is power.

The Family Physician (Your Coach)

Your family physician has a major role to play on your diabetes team; indeed, even if you have a diabetes specialist whom you see from time to time, your family doctor will still provide the great majority of your diabetes medical care. For this reason, if you are fortunate enough to live in one of the few communities remaining in Canada where you can actually choose your doctor, it is best to find a family physician that has a particular interest and expertise with diabetes. If you are unsure about this, simply ask them. If they do not feel that diabetes management is their forté, they may be able to recommend another doctor to help you.

Your family physician's responsibilities are far too numerous to list in their entirety (it would take many pages to itemize all the many tasks that these hard-working, dedicated doctors must do), but if we speak specifically in terms of your diabetes, here are just some of the things your family doctor will do:

✔ **Review any symptoms you may have developed:** In most cases, your family doctor should be your first point of contact if you have developed symptoms (for example, such things as mood problems, vaginal discharge, diarrhea, or numbness in your feet).

✔ **Review your blood glucose control:** We strongly recommend that you record your blood glucose readings in a logbook (see Chapter 6 for a detailed discussion of blood glucose record keeping) and that you review your numbers with your family doctor on a regular basis.

✔ **Examine you:** Routine components of your physical examination should include checking your blood pressure and pulse, feeling your thyroid, listening to your heart and lungs, and examining your feet for problems with your skin, circulation, or nerve function

✔ **Order screening studies:** There are a number of tests that your doctor should do from time to time, including checking your A1C, cholesterol, urine albumin/creatinine ratio, and so on.

✔ **Help organize your visits to other team members:** This includes things such as reviewing with you when you are due to see other team members — for example, your diabetes educators and your eye doctor — and, if necessary, arranging for visits to other providers, including your diabetes specialist and podiatrist.

Please note again that this list is not meant to be exhaustive and does not include the numerous things your family doctor helps you with, independent of your diabetes.

The Diabetes Specialist (Your General Manager)

Family physicians provide the great majority of diabetes care in Canada. Nonetheless, seeing a diabetes specialist from time to time is usually a good idea — especially if you have known complications from diabetes or if you have type 1 diabetes.

It is surprisingly difficult to define the term *diabetes specialist.* Sure, we can say it is "a doctor who specializes in diabetes," and although that would be accurate, it would still be incomplete. We can arbitrarily classify diabetes specialists into three groups:

✔ **Endocrinologists** (such as Alan): These are doctors who, after medical school, trained in internal medicine and then did additional training in endocrine ("hormone") disorders such as those affecting the pancreas (diabetes, for example), thyroid, and adrenal glands.

✔ **Internists** (such as Ian): These are doctors who, after medical school, trained in internal medicine and then usually tailored their practice to a particular area. In Ian's case this was diabetes. For other internal medicine specialists it is, for example, heart disease or high blood pressure.

✔ **Family Physicians:** This one may surprise you. Not many family physicians are diabetes specialists, but some are. These are doctors who, after medical school, trained in family medicine and then, because diabetes was a particular interest of theirs or because their community may not have had ready access to a diabetes specialist, or both, focused their practice on diabetes. We have given lectures to such family physicians and must admit we have felt that it just as well could have been *them* giving the talk.

The main reason to see a diabetes specialist is the greater likelihood that they will be — by virtue of the time they devote to this one topic — "on top of the literature," that they will know about new research findings and new and innovative forms of therapy.

Your diabetes specialist can assess your diabetes-related issues and develop a treatment plan that they can then share with other members of your health care team.

It is *essential* that your specialist send any reports to *all* relevant parties. Other-wise, using our previous hockey analogy, you and your specialist will be the only players on your team that are handling the puck. And that will make your other teammates less effective. Whenever you see your diabetes specialist, make a point of asking him or her to be sure to send a report to your family physician (*and* your diabetes educator). You shouldn't have to ask, but you do.

Your family physician, your diabetes, and you

As diabetes specialists we are indebted to family doctors. They provide the overwhelming majority of diabetes care in this country. Regrettably, the number of physicians choosing to make a career of family medicine is rapidly dwindling, making it harder and harder for Canadians to obtain basic medical care. Fewer family doctors means that those in this field have to look after more and more patients, which makes it that much harder for them to spend additional time with each individual in their practice. There is also a shortage of diabetes specialists, which puts additional work and responsibility on the shoulders of family physicians. The result is that numerous Canadians with diabetes (and people without diabetes too, of course) are not receiving all the care they require. All the more reason, therefore, that it is crucial for you to be an "informed consumer" and take on the responsibility of knowing what your health care requires.

Dr. Stewart Harris of London, Ontario, is a family physician. He is also the Chair of the Canadian Diabetes Association's Clinical and Scientific Section. Dr. Harris is a perfect example of why the label (be it "family physician," "internist," "endocrinologist," or whatever) does not necessarily tell the whole story. Indeed, given the realities of diabetes care in Canada, Dr. Harris says, "All family doctors are going to have to be diabetes specialists."

The Diabetes Educator (Your Trainer)

It is for good reason that a recent president of the American Diabetes Association once said, "Diabetes education is the single greatest advance ever made in diabetes care."

Although every member of your diabetes team is, in some way, shape, or form an educator, a diabetes *nurse* educator is typically the health care team member that provides the bulk of your initial and ongoing teaching. In Canada, diabetes educators generally have the initials *C.D.E.* ("certified *d*iabetes *e*ducator") after their names, however there are many excellent educators that do not have such certification. Diabetes educators are typically registered nurses that, after completing nursing school, have worked in hospitals or clinics and then went on to do further training to learn how to teach people about their diabetes.

Many dieticians are also certified diabetes educators (as are some pharmacists and, on occasion, some other type of health care provider) and, in addition to their role in teaching about proper nutrition, they can provide expert guidance about many other aspects of diabetes management; indeed, Claire Lightfoot, a dietician in Campbell River, British Columbia, was the recipient of the Canadian Diabetes Association's Diabetes Educator of the Year award for 2004.

A diabetes educator teaches you how to take your insulin or pills, how to test your blood glucose, and how to acquire many of the other skills you need. And that is just the beginning. They are invaluable resources, and if you have not met with a diabetes educator, you are truly missing out.

Diabetes educators' roles are progressively expanding. Not only do they continue to fulfill their traditional teaching role, they can also keep you up-to-date on new developments in diabetes therapy. Additionally, many educators now have the authority — as well they should — to test your A1C level (see Chapter 6), to help you adjust your insulin dosages, to adjust the dose of your oral hypoglycemic agents, to test your urine for evidence of kidney damage, and to measure your cholesterol levels. There are even some extraordinary (and extraordinarily *rare*) educators that carry pagers so that they can be contacted 24 hours a day if you are having problems.

If you have not met up with a diabetes educator, ask your doctor to refer you to one. If you have not seen your educator for some time, call to arrange a follow-up visit. What health professionals know about diabetes keeps changing, so why should you be left behind? Stay current; see your educator regularly. (If this sounds like a sales pitch, we offer no apologies. We think diabetes educators are wonderful — in case you hadn't noticed.)

The majority of doctors are fully aware of the essential role that diabetes educators and dietitians play and make a routine practice of referring their patients to them. (Trust us; it makes life a lot easier for the doctor to have other members of the health care team sharing the work!) Regrettably, there are some doctors who feel that diabetes educators and dietitians are superfluous and who will not send their patients to them. If you are placed in this unfortunate situation, ask your doctor to refer you anyhow. If he or she still refuses, call your local hospital diabetes clinic and ask if you can make an appointment without a doctor's referral.

The Dietitian (Your Energizer)

Remember the movie *Ghostbusters*? Well, when it comes to your nutrition plan (also called a "meal plan"), *who you gonna call?* Your dietitian.

Registered dieticians are the pros when it comes to assisting you with your nutrition. To be called a "registered dietitian" in Canada, a person must have official certification establishing that he or she has the appropriate credentials. In Canada, the initials *R.D.* appear after the name of certified dietitians.

What you eat (and drink) is central to your success with your diabetes. Eat poorly, and you will render many of the pills you are taking less effective. Your oral hypoglycemic agents will be less useful. Your blood pressure pills will not work as well. Your cholesterol medicine will be fighting an uphill battle. And so on.

Your dietitian is the most knowledgeable person when it comes to advising you about what you should eat. It would be a terrible disservice to them — and, more important, to you — to think of the dietitian's role as simply "putting you on a diet to lose weight." A dietitian can help you determine the best choice and quantity of foods, and he or she can help you determine the number of calories that your body requires.

If you have type 1 diabetes and are on an "intensified insulin" program, your dietitian can teach you how to keep track of your carbohydrates (called "carbohydrate counting"), which is often a highly effective means of achieving excellent blood glucose control. We discuss carbohydrate counting in Chapter 7.

A good dietitian will help you to create a nutrition plan that does the following:

 ✔ Stays flexible

 ✔ Takes into account your particular ethnic and cultural background, and meets your particular religious requirements (if any)

 ✔ Fits with your lifestyle

The importance of tailoring a diet to fit the individual can no be no better demonstrated than by the tale of two brothers that Ian had occasion to meet a couple of years ago. They were both teenagers and both also had type 1 diabetes. Bob was athletic and was captain of his hockey team. David, a year younger than his brother, couldn't have been more different. David could dismantle (and reassemble!) a car or a computer, but the only red line he knew about was the one on the tachometer. For the sake of convenience, the first time they were to meet with their dietitian they went together. The advice they received and the meal plans they took home were as different from one another as night and day. But the plans worked. To each his own (diet, that is!).

If you feel that the treatment plan your dietitian gives you is too rigid, that it is too out of keeping with your tastes, or that it is in some other way simply not realistic or practical, *do not* give up on the idea of proper nutrition therapy. Let your dietitian know of your concerns and he or she will likely be happy to work with you at creating a more appropriate meal plan.

The Eye Specialist (Your Cameraperson)

An eye doctor has special expertise in the detection and treatment of eye disease. There are two types of eye doctors — ophthalmologists and optometrists. We also look at the various types of eye disease for which you are at risk.

Eye damage from diabetes seldom causes symptoms until it is very advanced, so it *absolutely essential* that you see an eye doctor routinely — even if you have no problems with your sight!

Although your family doctor and your diabetes specialist may examine your eyes, an eye doctor has additional skills that you should avail yourself of.

Although spending inordinate time in doctors' waiting rooms is the stuff of legend, eye doctors' offices are particularly famous for this. Make sure you bring something to read when you go. Hmm . . . how about *Diabetes For Canadians For Dummies*? And you had best plan on doing your day's reading prior to going into the examining room, because when you see your eye specialist, he or she will dilate your pupils using eye drops. This can affect your vision for a few hours and may make it difficult for you to read, and, more important, may make it impossible for you to drive yourself home from your appointment. It would be wise, therefore, for you to bring someone with you to drive you home.

Sometimes the good deed of restoring vision leads to unexpected, negative consequences. One ophthalmologist told Alan that he restored the vision of a patient with diabetes, only to have the patient buy a gun and nearly shoot someone with whom he had a grievance!

The Pharmacist (Your Equipment Manager)

If you have diabetes, you are invariably going to be on medications to assist with our ultimate goal of keeping you healthy. Now, it may be that when you go to the pharmacy, your first thought is "oh heck, another errand." Okay, so going to a pharmacy isn't the highlight of your day (thankfully!). But what a great resource you have at your disposal in the form of your pharmacist.

Pharmacists have expertise in medicines, so when you pick up your prescriptions, you have a golden opportunity to become an informed consumer. Here are some of the things that your pharmacist should review with you:

✔ The names of your medicines

✔ The dosages of your medicines

✔ How often you are to take your medicines

✔ What time you should take your medicines (for example, many cholesterol medicines work best if taken in the evening)

✔ What route you are to take your medicines (oral, vaginal, topical, and so on)

✔ Whether you should take your medicines with food or on an empty stomach

✔ Whether it is safe for you to consume alcohol (Some people have bad reactions if they ingest alcohol while on sulfonylurea oral hypoglycemic agents.).

✔ Whether there are any possible interactions between your different medicines (For example, thyroid pills don't get absorbed as effectively if you take them at the same time as calcium pills.)

✔ What adverse effects ("side effects") the medicines can cause.

A good pharmacist will not simply hand your pills to you with a piece of paper (listing 50 side effects) stapled to your bag and say goodbye. A good pharmacist will sit down with you and not only explain the items listed above, but also review with you *how likely* it is that you will experience the different side effects. Without a pharmacist's help, as you read through the lengthy list of all the bad things that the medicines can do you will not be truly informed. You will simply be scared. And *that* is not effective counselling.

If you are on several (or more) different medicines, ask your pharmacist to prepare a list of your medications that you can keep in your wallet or purse. This list should include the names, doses, and frequency of your drugs. Keeping track of when to take medicines can be very difficult. Your pharmacist may be able to help you out by packaging your medicines in a container where they are laid out by day of week and time of day.

The Foot Doctor (Your Sole Mate)

The foot doctor (*podiatrist*) is your best source of help with the minor and some of the major foot problems that you may encounter. He or she can assist you with such problems as toenails that are hard to cut, bothersome corns and calluses, and difficulties with excessively dry or cracked skin. If you have areas of your feet that undergo excessive pressure as you walk, a foot doctor can also help fit you with special insoles called orthotics, which more evenly distribute the forces upon your feet.

The longer we are in practice as diabetes specialists, the more we have come to rely on and use the expertise that podiatrists have to offer. They truly are the experts when it comes to helping you keep your feet healthy.

Not all podiatry services are covered by provincial health care plans. Before you meet with your podiatrist, you might want to call ahead to find out what charges you may expect.

Your Family and Friends (Your Fans and Cheerleaders)

Okay, so the 1985 Oilers likely would have done just fine, thank you very much, even if they didn't have a single fan in the stands. But they were the exceptions. For the rest of us, it is essential to have people rooting for us as we deal with the trials and tribulations of life. And this is especially true if you are living with a health issue such as diabetes.

Your fans and cheerleaders are the people you live with, eat with, and play with. Your family and friends can be a tremendous source of support, but for them to help you, they will need your guidance. For example, you can teach them what to look for if you become hypoglycemic (see Chapter 4). And you can ask them to avoid eating indiscriminately in your presence. Following your diet is challenging enough; you certainly don't need your family exposing you to constant temptation. Your family or friends can also become your exercise partners. Sticking to a program is a lot easier when a partner is counting on you to show up to work out.

It is often a good idea to have someone accompany you when you see a member of your health care team. (This is especially true if you are meeting the dietitian and you are not the main food preparer at home.) A lot of information is going to be communicated, and an extra set of ears is helpful.

If you do plan to bring an extra set of ears with you to your doctor's appointment, be sure to ask your physician ahead of time if it is okay to bring this person in. There may, on occasion, be some issues that should be discussed in private before your friend or relative joins you. (Important conversations about, say, sexual dysfunction, likely would not take place if you have your daughter or son in the room as you are speaking to your doctor.)

Let people who are important to you know about your diabetes. Showing them this chapter might be a good way to introduce them to their important supporting role.

In this chapter we look at the central players on your diabetes team, but it is important to recognize that there are many other teammates who may be asked to take a face-off from time to time. These include, among others, hospital emergency room staff, heart specialists, neurologists, gastroenterologists ("stomach doctors"), social workers, dentists, psychologists, and psychiatrists.

Chapter 6

Monitoring Your Blood Glucose Control

....

In This Chapter

▶ Understanding the whys and wherefores of blood glucose monitoring

▶ Choosing a glucose meter

▶ Testing your blood

▶ Knowing when to test

▶ Knowing your targets

▶ Assessing longer term control with an A1C

....

*Y*ou're among the most fortunate people with diabetes who have ever lived. We have nutrition therapy, we have exercise techniques, we have prescription medicines, and we have non-prescription products. And to make sure that we are reaching our goals, we have the benefit of testing equipment to help us monitor our progress. Sure, it's a bit of a bother and will cost some money, but, hey, you're worth it.

Most of the products and treatments we cover in this chapter were not available even 20 years ago. And the new products coming along will knock your socks off (but put them back on because you should not go barefoot).

Testing with a Glucose Meter

In earlier chapters we discuss the bad things that can happen if you are exposed to elevated blood glucose. In this chapter, you discover all you need to know about how to monitor your blood glucose levels.

"Why monitor?" you might ask. "After all, my doctor can just send me to the lab for a blood test when I need it."

True enough. Your doctor *can* just send you to the lab for a blood test when you need it. But that would mean visiting the lab *every* day. Surely, you have better things to do with your time.

Why you should test

Have you even gotten dressed in the dark only to find out as you were heading out the door that your socks were mismatched or the blue pants you put on were actually black or your red purse was actually brown? You probably either made a mad dash back inside to re-dress, or you just headed out, hoping that your gaffe would not be noticed. Well, not monitoring your blood glucose levels is like getting dressed in the dark every day.

If you are not testing your blood, you will never know:

- ✔ If your nutrition ("diet") plan (see Chapter 7) is helping your glucose control
- ✔ If your exercise program is improving your glucose levels
- ✔ If your oral hypoglycemic agents or insulin doses need to be changed
- ✔ If your recent illness, such as a chest infection, is making your glucose readings dangerously high

Basically, you will be in the dark, without guidance, and equally important, without feedback.

But what if your readings are poor? "Why do I want to be frustrated by always seeing crummy readings?" you might ask. And you would be perfectly justified in asking this. At least, you would be perfectly justified if there were no way to improve things. But there are *always* ways to improve things. So if your readings are not good, it is time for you to meet with your diabetes educator and dietitian to see if your lifestyle plan needs adjusting. And to call your family doctor (or diabetes specialist if you are in regular contact with one) to have your oral hypoglycemic agents or insulin therapy reviewed.

There is a tendency for people with diabetes to look at a record of their glucose readings as a report card, keeping constant score and noting whether they have passed or failed. That is understandable, but terribly inappropriate. Your glucose readings are not meant to judge you or your efforts. Your readings are being done to serve as an aid — a tool — to help you and your team know when changes to your therapy are in order. And if your readings are good, they serve as a nice source of positive feedback.

How often should you test?

How often you test is determined by three factors: the kind of diabetes you have, the kind of treatment you are using, and the level of stability of your blood glucose. As you can tell, this is not a "one size fits all" issue. The Canadian Diabetes Association (CDA) recommends the following:

- ✔ **If you have type 1 diabetes:** Test at least three times daily (and, periodically, overnight). Many situations require more frequent testing to achieve desired blood glucose levels.

- ✔ **If you have type 2 diabetes:** Test at least once daily if you are being treated with oral hypoglycemic agents or insulin. Many situations require more frequent testing to achieve desired blood glucose levels.

- ✔ **Tests should include both before-meal and two-hour post-meal readings.** (Tricky indeed if you are testing only once — or even three times — daily!) Well, what the CDA means is that you should vary the timing of your tests from one day to the next, not that you need to test before and 2 hours after meals *every* day. We will look at some possible testing schedules in a moment.

In our experience, the more you test, the more information and feedback you have, and, ultimately, the better you do. For this reason we would encourage you to focus on the "at least" wording of the CDA guidelines and aim to test considerably more often than the minimum recommendations. We have found the following schedule to work very well (note that this schedule assumes your overall control is both very good and very stable; if it is not, you should be testing *even more*):

✔ **If your treatment consists of lifestyle measures alone,** test *once* daily, varying the timing of your reading so that over the span of a week or two you will have values from before and after each of your meals.

✔ **If you are taking oral hypoglycemic agents,** test *twice* daily:

- Before breakfast, *and*

- Vary the time of the other test (sometimes do it before your other meals and sometimes 2 hours after your meals).

✔ **If you are an adult taking insulin once or twice a day,** test *twice* daily:

- Before breakfast, *and*

- Vary the time of the other test (sometimes do it before your other meals, sometimes 2 hours after your meals, and *sometimes at bedtime*).

✔ **If you are an adult taking insulin three or four times a day (or a child or adolescent taking insulin any number of times a day),** test *four to seven* times daily:

- Before each meal, *and*

- 2 hours after some meals (you may wish to rotate so that one day you test after breakfast, the next day after lunch, and the next day after dinner), *and*

- Every night at bedtime, *and*

- *Occasionally at about 3 am* (to make sure you are not having low overnight readings that have not been awakening you).

✔ **If you have gestational diabetes** treated with lifestyle measures alone, test before and 2 hours after your breakfast.

✔ **If you are pregnant and have pre-existing diabetes or if you have gestational diabetes treated with insulin,** test *six to seven* times per day (before and 2 hours after each meal and again at bedtime if your bedtime is 4 or more hours after your dinner).

Never fall into the trap of assuming that if you feel well, your blood glucose levels *must* be good and therefore you do not need to test. The truth is, your blood glucose level can be twice (or more) normal and you may not have a single symptom, while all the while your body is being irreversibly damaged.

As you can tell from this list, the frequency of testing is directly related to how often you need the information to make decisions about your care. If you are being treated with lifestyle measures alone, getting feedback once per day is usually enough to let you know how effective your treatment plan is, whereas if you are on an intensified insulin program, you should test much more often to know what insulin dose to administer.

Most everyone has periods of time where they get fed up with testing, testing, testing. Don't feel guilty if you feel this way; it is perfectly normal. And if you do happen to go through periods of time where you are not testing nearly as much as you should, there's no need to berate yourself about it. Just grab hold of your meter and get back into the routine.

Mr. Pereira was a middle-aged man with type 2 diabetes who had come to Ian's office for a consultation. Ian asked him how his blood glucose control was, and Mr. Pereira replied, "It was 7.4 today." Ian asked him if he had any other readings to share. "Sure; it was 9.3 last month so it's getting better." Ian explained to his patient that glucose control varies not only month to month, but day to day and even meal to meal, so knowing two readings taken a month apart tells us virtually nothing about how control is or what trend it is following. Hearing this explanation, Mr. Pereira, a math teacher, asked if he could borrow Ian's calculator, and, a moment later, announced, "Gee, Doctor, now I get it. I've told you what my readings were for a total of 2 minutes out of the past 43,200 minutes. That's not even five one-thousandths of 1 percent of my readings. *No wonder* that doesn't tell you much." Couldn't have said it better ourselves.

How do you perform a test?

Just like any test, a blood glucose test requires some basic supplies:

> ✔ **Lancet:** If you happen to be like us, the notion of intentionally wounding yourself is most definitely not your idea of a good time. Well, you need not despair because

obtaining a blood sample is a nearly painless procedure. In order to prick yourself you use a small, sharp, disposable *lancet*.

✔ **Lancet holder:** Your lancet fits into this spring-loaded holder, and when you push the release button, the lancet springs out and pokes your finger.

✔ **Test strip:** This is the small disposable strip onto which you place your drop of blood.

✔ **Blood glucose meter:** This is the device that figures out how much glucose is in your blood sample. We'll talk more about these neat gadgets in a moment.

✔ **"Sharps" container:** This is a small box into which you place your used lancets. You can pick up a sharps container from your drugstore. When the container is full, seal it and bring it back to the drugstore for proper disposal.

Though you may be apprehensive about pricking yourself to obtain a drop of blood, rest assured that you will be far more relaxed than a man in his 20s that Ian knew of. This man was converting to a religion that required a ritual drop of blood to be obtained from the end part of his penis. The man lay down and the appropriate part of his anatomy was exposed. A physician was called into the room to obtain the drop of blood. The physician, a twinkle in his eye, looked down at the anxious man and said he need not worry, the procedure would be over in a minute. "I've got a new medical instrument I just obtained when I was travelling overseas," the doctor said. "It will work perfectly," he added as he reached behind him and brought into full view a Samurai sword! (P.S. The procedure actually did go ahead — the mischievous doctor using a tiny needle in lieu of the sword.)

Now, let's look at the, ahem, more conventional steps in obtaining a blood sample:

1. **Wash your hands (or at least your finger):** Although you do not need to prepare your site — or your psyche — with alcohol, you need to make sure your finger (or arm if you are using an "alternate-site meter," which we discuss in the next section) is clean.

2. **Obtain a blood sample:** Insert a lancet into the lancet holder, press it against the *side* of your fingertip, and

activate the trigger. In an instant, you will see a tiny drop of blood appear. It does not hurt much at all, but to make it hurt even less you can:

- Use a lancet holder that allows you to adjust the depth of penetration. An example is the Softclix Lancing Device.

- Avoid re-using your lancets since they dull quickly. (It's okay to use the same one a few times, but not more than that.)

- Change fingers often or, quite the opposite, stick to the side of the same finger and you will find that once you have built up a small callus it hurts less to draw blood from that site.

- Take blood from an "alternate site" such as your forearm. (To do this you will need an "alternate-site meter.")

3. **Apply the end of the glucose-measuring strip to the blood:** Only a tiny drop of blood is required, but it still has to be sufficient to cover the marked area on the strip. Most strips are designed to draw up the blood in the same way that a strip of paper towel, when dipped into water, draws up the water (a process called "capillary action," in case you were wondering).

4. **Presto, you're done:** Most modern meters will then quickly display your result.

If you have difficulty obtaining a sufficient quantity of blood, try one or more of the following:

- ✔ Warm your finger with warm water.

- ✔ Let your arm hang down at your side for a minute before you test.

- ✔ Hold your finger about 1.5 centimetres (about half an inch) from the tip and squeeze — but only once, as repeated squeezing can interfere with the test's accuracy.

How a blood glucose meter works

Earlier glucose meters relied on a colour change that appeared on the test strips and that was proportional to your blood glucose level. The new meters use a different process to analyze your blood. They measure an electrical potential that is created when the glucose in your blood sample reacts with reagents (glucose oxidase and potassium ferricyanide) on the electrode of the test strip. This reaction generates electrons that produce an electrical current. The higher your glucose level, the greater the current.

If ever you find that your test result is far lower than you expect, this may be because you had insufficient blood on the strip (this can give falsely low readings). If your blood glucose meter tells you that your reading is, for example, 2.8 mmol/L and you had expected a 12.8 mmol/L, re-test yourself. On the other hand, you can obtain falsely elevated readings if the test strips have been exposed to high humidity or high temperature. Be sure to read the package insert that came with your strips to familiarize yourself with the instructions (and precautions) made by the manufacturer.

Incidentally, when it comes to used lancets, remember the old adage: Neither a borrower nor a lender be. The only time you should share your blood is when you are donating to Canadian Blood Services. Similarly, because a meter invariably gets a little blood on it (and hence, can be a source of infection), you should not share your meter.

How Do You Choose a Meter?

So many meters are on the market that you may be confused about which one to use. One consideration that should play little or no part in your choice of a meter is the cost, since with rebates, promotions, trade-ins (and, most of all, because the companies are happy to sell their machines at a loss in order to get you to buy their strips), you will find *almost* every meter you look at to be quite inexpensive and competitively priced. Because the meters are so cheap and because the manufacturers replace them with better ones so frequently, it is a good idea to get a new meter every year or two, to make sure that you have the "latest and greatest" device.

Another non-consideration is the accuracy of the various machines. All are accurate to a degree acceptable for managing your diabetes. Keep in mind, though, that they do not have the accuracy of laboratory equipment. (If ever you are experimenting with your machine and test your blood twice within a minute or two, you may find your readings vary by 10 to 15 percent. This is not because your blood glucose level has changed that amount in a matter of seconds; it is simply that the machines are not perfect.)

Although the meters are cheap, the test strips are anything but. Typically they are about a dollar per strip (ouch!), regardless of which meter you are using. If you shop around, however, you will find that some drugstores sell them for significantly less than others.

 Some provinces and territories will subsidize the cost of your blood glucose strips. For more information you can contact your provincial or territorial government or the CDA. (Excellent information is available on the CDA Web site, www.diabetes. ca. Click Advocacy, then click the link entitled Financial Coverage Charts for Diabetes Supplies and Medication.)

Capillary versus venous glucose levels

When you test with a finger-prick sample, you are obtaining what is termed a "capillary" blood sample, whereas when a lab takes blood from your arm they are obtaining a "venous" blood sample. The glucose level in a venous sample is typically about 15 percent higher than a capillary sample. This would make your meter's results misleadingly low, so the testing equipment has been designed to correct for this.

Since the machines are similar in price, similar in accuracy, and similar in terms of the costs for their strips, your purchase decision should be based on other factors:

✔ Whether you like products with "bells and whistles" or prefer those that are "plain and simple."

✔ If your eyesight is poor, you will want to make sure the display is easily readable or, if that is not sufficient, you may wish to purchase a meter that can connect with a voice synthesizer. (The SureStep and OneTouch meters can connect to a "voice box" sold by Auto Control Medical — 800-461-0991 — for approximately $400. This synthesizer is truly amazing, but you will have to put up with — how can we say this kindly — the voice of a particularly assertive gentleman.)

✔ If you are likely to be testing in the dark you will want to select a meter that has backlighting. There is even a meter that is itself glow-in-the-dark (the Precision Xtra).

✔ If you want to test from "alternate sites" such as your forearm, there are now meters designed to allow this (such as the OneTouch Ultra and the Freestyle).

✔ You will want to make sure the meter is not too bulky (seldom an issue with current meters), or, conversely, too small to fit comfortably in your hand. For example, the brand new "FreeStyle mini" is an amazingly compact meter which will make it a great choice for some people and not a good choice for others.

✔ Some strips are larger than others. If you have a hard time holding onto very small objects, you may wish to choose a meter (such as the AccuSoft Advantage) that uses larger strips.

✔ You will have to decide how much memory you need in a machine. They can vary considerably in terms of how many readings they store. If you are keeping a written logbook — which we recommend — this is not a particularly important feature, but if you are not keeping a logbook, a memory is a good thing to have (in a meter, not to mention in our heads!). The OneTouch UltraSmart has an excellent, though not perfect, way of presenting records stored in its memory.

✔ If you have type 1 diabetes, it would be a good idea to use a meter that also tests for ketones, such as the Precision Xtra.

✔ You may find it more convenient to have a device that can hold multiple test strips. Examples include the DEX2 and the Accu-Chek Compact.

✔ If you like the idea of being able to download your readings onto your computer so you can graph (and print) them, you will want to buy a meter that has this capacity. Bear in mind that you will likely encounter an additional charge for the connecting cable.

✔ If you are using insulin, NovoNordisk and Lifescan have teamed up to make a nice product called the InDuo. It has two components — a meter and an insulin pen device — that fit together into a fairly small package.

✔ If time is of the essence, you will want to have a lightning-fast machine. Depending on the machine, it can take from 5 to 30 seconds to process a sample and display the result.

Alternate-site glucose readings are not reliable if they are obtained when your blood glucose level is rapidly rising or falling. For this reason, you should not rely on alternate-site tests if you are doing a blood glucose test within 2 hours of eating, nor should you use an alternate site test if you suspect you are hypoglycemic.

You will save much time, energy, and aggravation by speaking to your diabetes educator before you buy a meter. Not only can he or she show you the latest meters and point out their pros and cons, but also, more important, *they know you* and will be able to help you select a meter that meets your particular needs.

If you would like to do some of your own research, you can find (far from impartial) information regarding meters by going to the different manufacturers' Web sites or by calling them. Here are the main manufacturers in the Canadian market, their current products, Web sites, and phone numbers:

Table 6-1	Manufacturers and Meters	
Manufacturer	*Product*	*Contact information*
Abbott Diabetes Care	FreeStyle FreeStyle Mini Precision Xtra	www.abbottdiabetescare.com **888-519-6890**
Bayer	Ascensia Breeze Ascensia Contour Ascensia DEX2 Ascensia Elite Ascensia Elite XL	www.bayer.ca **800-268-1432**
Becton-Dickson	BD Logic Latitude Diabetes Management System The Link	www.bddiabetes.com **800-268-5430**
Lifescan	OneTouch Ultra OneTouch UltraSmart OneTouch SureStep	www.lifescancanada.com **800-663-5521**
Lifescan/ NovoNordisk	InDuo	www.novonordisk.ca **800-465-4334**
Roche	AccuSoft Advantage Accu-Check Aviva Accu-Chek Compact	www.rochecanada.com **800-363-7949**

How Should You Record Your Results?

Ian recalls going for a haircut a few years back (when he used to have to go more often) only to find his barber profoundly upset. "What's the matter?" Ian asked, to which his barber replied that he could not find his scissors. "Why not just use somebody else's?" Ian innocently asked. His barber immediately stopped his searching and looked at Ian with disbelief. "Use somebody else's? Would you use somebody else's wife?" And that just about sums up most diabetes specialists' opinions about how glucose readings should be recorded. We are very particular and we each have our own preferences.

So then, we *could* show you many different ways of recording your results, or we could just show you the best way, which, ahem, just happens to be Ian's way!

The first thing you need to do is to obtain a logbook. You can find these at your pharmacy, at your diabetes education centre, and at your diabetes specialist's office. Your family doctor may also have them. Each page in your logbook should be laid out like this:

	Blood Glucose Levels							Insulin Injections					
Date	Breakfast		Lunch		Dinner		Bedtime	Other	Insulin Type	Units Taken				Notes
	Before	After	Before	After	Before	After				Breakfast	Lunch	Dinner	Bedtime	

Figure 6-1: Logbook format.

Of course, if you are not on insulin the right hand side of the page will go unused.

Most logbooks, alas, do not have this particular format. If you are unable to find a book with this layout, you can download (for free) similar pages from Ian's Web site (www.ianblumer.ca).

The one shortcoming with this layout is, potentially, insufficient space for you to write in the Notes column (where you might want to write things such as "birthday party" or "missed snack" to remind you later on of some event that had occurred that might explain a high or low reading). If you need more space, you can always create your own sheet on a piece of paper (which you could photocopy) or with a spreadsheet program such as Excel.

Using this layout allows you to quickly assess your overall blood glucose *patterns, trends,* and *averages* for a given time of day. To illustrate what we mean, let's have a look at two different ways of recording your readings.

The following table is the typical way that a log is kept or that a machine's memory displays results (although a machine would display the time of day, not the meal of the day). The following readings are pre-meal values:

Table 6-2	Blood Glucose Readings Listed Chronologically
Time of Reading	*Blood Glucose Level*
Breakfast	12.6
Lunch	4.1
Dinner	14.7
Bedtime	5.6
Breakfast	11.7
Lunch	5.2
Dinner	12.1
Bedtime	7.0
Breakfast	10.0
Lunch	5.9
Dinner	11.9
Bedtime	4.0
Breakfast	9.9
Lunch	4.2
Dinner	14.4
Bedtime	4.4
Breakfast	11.1
Lunch	6.3
Dinner	12.2
Bedtime	5.1

If you were to record your readings like this, you would likely feel that your glucose values were "all over the place" (or, as Ian often hears, "my sugars are up and down like a toilet seat") and you would likely be feeling frustrated by what you concluded were very inconsistent values. Although your conclusion would be perfectly understandable, you might be surprised to see that if we look at your readings from a different perspective, they could be thought of as being remarkably consistent. Let's take those same readings and chart them differently.

Table 6-3 Blood Glucose Readings Listed by Time of Day

Breakfast	Lunch	Dinner	Bedtime
12.6	4.1	14.7	5.6
11.7	5.2	12.1	7.0
10.0	5.9	11.9	4.0
9.9	4.2	14.4	4.4
11.1	6.3	12.2	5.1

Now, scan the columns from top to bottom. Aha! You will see that your readings at any given time of day are remarkably similar. You are consistently too high at breakfast, consistently normal at lunch, consistently too high at dinner, and consistently normal at bedtime.

The memory on a blood glucose meter does not allow for this type of instant overview, and hence is almost always inferior to using a logbook. (The only meter that comes close is the OneTouch UltraSmart, but even that one does not give as complete a picture as those old and trusted tools: pen and paper.)

This is of great importance because now that we have identified your blood glucose patterns, we can adjust your therapy accordingly. For example, if you were on insulin therapy, we would know that you need more bedtime insulin to bring down your breakfast blood glucose and more lunchtime insulin to reduce your suppertime readings. We could have figured this out from the first table, but it would have been much more difficult and time consuming.

TIP

If you are using an insulin pump you will need an even more detailed log book; a good one can be found at Rick Mendosa's Web site (www.mendosa.com/logsheet.pdf).

What Is Your Glucose Target?

The Canadian Diabetes Association (CDA) guidelines recommend that *most* adults with type 1 or type 2 diabetes aim for the following readings:

	Before meals	*2 hours after meals*
Target	4.0-7.0 mmol/L	5.0-10.0 mmol/L
Normal level	4.0-6.0 mmol/L	5.0-8.0 mmol/L

If you can do so safely, target the normal level. Here are some of the things that might make it unsafe for you to aim for normal levels:

✔ You have other health problems that make it too dangerous to risk any hypoglycemia.

✔ You have *irreversible* problems with hypoglycemia unawareness.

✔ When you try to have readings in this range, you experience excessively *frequent* hypoglycemia.

✔ Your life expectancy is such that you are at low risk of developing diabetes-related long-term complications.

No one with diabetes has glucose readings that are always within target. Indeed, having two-thirds of your readings within target is a wonderful accomplishment. And remember that to achieve (or to even come close to achieving) your targets will require a concerted and ongoing effort on behalf of your diabetes team. (And remember, *you* are the first star on this team.)

WARNING!

It can be very difficult to consistently achieve target blood glucose values and, for some people, it may simply not be possible. If you and your health care team have worked hard at reaching these goals but have not been able to achieve them it is essential that you not feel that all is lost. The reason for this is simple; although fantastic blood glucose readings are our goal, any improvement in your blood glucose control will help keep you free of complications from your diabetes. (See the following discussion on A1C testing.)

Testing for Longer-Term Control with an A1C

As Ian's mathematician discovered (in an anecdote earlier in this chapter), individual blood glucose tests are great for telling us how you're doing at a specific moment in time, but they do not give us the big picture. Frequent blood glucose measurements help, but even then, they only provide a series of snapshots of your glucose levels. So what we need is a test that gives an estimate of your *overall* control over a longer period of time. And that is precisely what we can determine from a test called an A1C. As the sidebar in this section discusses, your A1C level is a measure of how much glucose has become attached to your red blood cells over the preceding three to four months.

Knowing your A1C is crucial because the likelihood of your developing microvascular complications (that is, eye, kidney, and nerve damage) is directly related to your A1C. A normal A1C is 6 or less. An A1C of 7 is good and puts you at quite low risk for microvascular damage. An A1C of 9 or higher is poor and puts you at much greater risk. An A1C that is too high is an alarm to you and your health care team that your control needs to be improved. If you can drop your A1C by even 1 percent you will substantially decrease your risk of microvascular complications. In one landmark study — the "DCCT" — it was found that reducing the A1C from 8 down to about 7 (equivalent to a reduction in average blood glucose of only 2 mmol/L) resulted in an astounding 40 to 50 percent lower risk of retinopathy progression.

You may come across other terms for A1C, including "hemoglobin A1C," "glycosylated hemoglobin," or "glycohemoglobin." You may also come across it abbreviated as HbA1C or HgbA1C. These all mean the same thing. Also you may find an A1C level written as a number ("9," for example) or as a percentage ("9 %," for example); both of these are correct and mean the same thing.

After you have had your A1C tested, be sure you contact your doctor (or educator, if he or she is the one that requested the test) to find out the result!

The A1C does not replace blood glucose meter testing; it is *complementary* to it. Since the A1C represents an overall estimate of your blood glucose control, it does not tell us how many highs and lows you may be having. Your average glucose level may be good even though half your readings are too low and the other half too high. It's sort of like having one foot in ice water and the other in boiling water and saying "on average, I feel fine."

The following table shows what the average blood glucose levels are (over the preceding three to four months) for a given A1C:

Table 6-4   A1C with Corresponding Average Blood Glucose Level

A1C	Average blood glucose level (in mmol/L)
5	5.5
6	7.5
7	9.5
8	11.5
9	13.5
10	15.5
11	17.5
12	19.5

As the table demonstrates, the higher your A1C, the higher your blood glucose levels have been running. The lower your A1C, the lower your recent blood glucose levels. The Canadian Diabetes Association recommends that your A1C level be tested every three months. (If you are pregnant it will need to be checked more often.)

As you can see, your A1C reading is *not* the same as your average blood glucose. This is commonly misunderstood. (For example, an A1C of 8.0 does *not* mean that your average blood glucose level is 8.0 mmol/L; it actually corresponds to average readings of 11.5 mmol/L.)

The Canadian Diabetes Association (CDA) guidelines recommend that *most* people with type 1 or type 2 diabetes aim for an A1C of 7 percent or less (normal is 6 percent or less for most laboratories). If it can be safely achieved (see the earlier discussion about why it might be unsafe), your goal is to have an A1C in the normal range.

As long as you use your glucose meter frequently, your A1C result will likely be as anticipated. When it isn't (for example, if your meter's average was 7.0 mmol/L yet your A1C was 10), you and your health care team will need to figure out why. The most common reason for this is that your readings are up when you are not testing and therefore you would not be aware of the elevations. If your readings have this sort of discrepancy, try testing more often and at times you haven't been testing (including overnight). On occasion an A1C level is affected by other substances in the blood or by anemia. If your physician suspects this, he or she can contact the laboratory to discuss this possibility.

Apart from going to the lab to have them take blood from your arm, there are two other ways to check an A1C. Some diabetes centres have a desktop machine that can process a fingerprick sample in 6 minutes so that you (and they) will know your result while you are there for your visit. The cost is usually about $10 per test. There is also a disposable test kit for home use called A1C Now. It is expensive, though, at about $50 per test.

How A1C works

Within red blood cells there is a protein called hemoglobin. Hemoglobin carries oxygen around the body, delivering it to where it is needed to assist with various chemical reactions that are taking place. Hemoglobin is constantly exposed to the glucose within the blood and becomes permanently attached to it. It attaches in several different ways, and the total of all the hemoglobin attached to glucose is called *glycohemoglobin.* The largest fraction, two-thirds of the glycohemoglobin, is in a form called hemoglobin A1C. This is the easiest form to measure. The rest of the hemoglobin is made up of hemoglobins A1a and A1b. The more glucose in the blood, the more glycohemoglobin forms. Hemoglobin is destroyed when the red blood cell that contains it dies. This occurs after the red blood cell has been in existence for about 120 days or so. Because glycohemoglobin remains in the blood for that length of time, it is a reflection of the glucose control over that entire time period and not just the second that a single glucose test reflects.

Chapter 7

Lifestyles That Will Help You Become Richly and Famously Healthy

● ●

In This Chapter

▶ Adjusting your diet to enhance your health

▶ Counting on carbohydrates

▶ Using the power of proteins

▶ Getting the facts on fatty foods

▶ Looking at the Atkins Diet: Is it for you?

▶ Finding out about the glycemic index

▶ Adding alcohol

▶ Determining if you are overweight

▶ Accomplishing weight loss

● ●

*L*anguage specialists claim that the five sweetest phrases in the English language are:

✔ I love you.

✔ Dinner is served.

✔ All is forgiven.

✔ Sleep until noon.

✔ Keep the change.

To that, most people would certainly add, "You've lost weight."

If you have diabetes and you are overweight and sedentary — and that is true of the great majority of people with type 2 diabetes — appropriate nutrition, weight loss, and exercise are your tickets to success. You have more power at your disposal than any drug that any doctor can dispense to you.

It may well be that you look back at your high school grad photos and point out to your children or grandchildren how slim and trim you were way back when exercise was not a chore, but a matter of routine. Perhaps it was not long thereafter that family and work commitments appeared, followed in short order by some excess weight around your middle. And once your lifestyle had changed, maybe you were like millions of your fellow Canadians and simply could never find the time or enthusiasm to get on track with exercise and shedding the extra kilograms you had acquired.

But the wonderful thing is, you are not too late. You are *never* too late. Whether you are 25 or 85, you can still make changes in your lifestyle to enhance your health. And you do not have to feel intimidated by this. The changes do not have to occur overnight. And the changes do not have to be "all or none," because any change is a change for the better.

And we can promise you that the changes you have to make are not quite so intimidating as those recommended by Hippocrates, the renowned physician of ancient times, who said "obese people should perform hard work, eat only once a day, take no baths, and walk naked as much as possible."

This chapter will provide you with the key information you need to follow a healthy lifestyle. We will review the role of "diet" therapy — we prefer to call it nutrition therapy. And as for walking naked as much as possible, well, if you choose to, remember to at least wear shoes and socks!

Diabetes and Nutrition — A Recipe for Success

Wanda B. Thinner (okay, we admit it; we changed the name), age 46, was recently diagnosed with type 2 diabetes. When the diagnosis was made, her doctor put her on some pills to reduce her blood glucose, but they were not helping and she continued to be bothered by excessive thirst and urination. When she was referred to Alan, she had a blood glucose of 13 mmol/L. She was 165 centimetres (5 feet 5 inches) tall and weighed 75 kilograms (165lb). Although she had been told by her doctor that she had to lose weight, no further instructions had been given. Alan immediately arranged for her to meet with a registered dietitian — and diabetes educator — and Mrs. Thinner started a lifestyle treatment program that included a meal plan based on the principles in this chapter. She worked hard over the next few months and successfully lost 9 kilograms (20 lb), which she subsequently kept off. Her blood glucose levels came down to the range of 6 to 7 mmol/L and her readings stayed there even after she stopped taking pills. She felt the best she had in years. Mrs. Thinner was yet another prime example of how pills are second-rate diabetes therapy compared to the impact of lifestyle treatment.

One of the single greatest obstacles to effective lifestyle therapy is expecting too much too soon. If you need to lose 23 kilograms (50 lb) and after a month you have lost only 2 kilograms (4 lb) you may start to feel frustrated, as if you are "never going to get there." But we wouldn't suggest for a second that you have not had success. You would have had *great success!* Diabetes is a long-term disease. Achieving your target weight does not have to occur overnight, or even over weeks or months. Slow and steady surely does win the weight-loss race. In fact, if you lose weight too quickly (see later in this chapter) you will be more likely to regain it. Before we talk further about techniques to help you lose weight, it would be a good idea to first look at the fundamental elements that make for a healthy nutrition plan.

 Nothing is so likely to frustrate your efforts at following proper nutrition therapy as trying to figure it out without professional help. We would strongly recommend that in addition to reading this chapter, you see a professional dietitian that has expertise in helping people with diabetes. If your doctor has not referred you to one, as soon as you finish reading this chapter, pick up the phone, call your doctor's office, and ask them to book you an appointment. You'll be glad you did.

The key ingredients

Our diets are made up primarily of carbohydrates, proteins, and fats. These basic groups are rounded out by the other things we need to consume to survive, including minerals, vitamins, and, of course, water. And, for most of us, our diets also include some degree of alcohol and, often, non-nutritive sweeteners. Despite what Ian's boys insist, cookie-dough ice cream *does not* constitute a separate and indispensable food group.

The Canadian Diabetes Association (CDA) recommends that people with diabetes follow Canada's Guidelines for Healthy Eating (you can find it online at www.hc-sc.gc.ca):

- Enjoy a variety of foods.
- Emphasize cereals, breads and other whole grain products, fruits and vegetables.
- Choose lower-fat dairy products, leaner meats and food prepared with little or no fat.
- Achieve and maintain a healthy body weight by enjoying regular physical activity and healthy eating.
- Limit salt, alcohol and caffeine.

The CDA guidelines also recommend that your diet be divided (based on energy, or calories) as follows:

- Carbohydrate: 50–55%
- Protein: 15–20%
- Fat: less than 30%

The number of calories contained in 1 gram is

- Carbohydrate: 4 calories
- Protein: 4 calories
- Fat: 9 calories

Of course, you and your dietitian will have to determine the best diet for you based on your particular needs. Your diet will include not only the best food choices for you, but also, the appropriate number of calories you should consume.

With unrestricted calories you could limit your carbohydrates to 50 percent of your diet and still have enough energy to power a Boeing 747.

Technically speaking, there is a "calorie" and there is a "Calorie" and there is a kilocalorie (1000 calories equals 1 *Calorie* equals 1 *kilo*calorie). However, almost no one speaks of kilocalories in normal, day-to-day discourse, and it's a chore to capitalize the "c" every time, so we use the conventional "calorie" whenever we are talking about nutrition issues. Sure, it is not perfectly scientific to do so, but we won't tell if you won't. (Also, you may come across the term *kilojoules*. One *Calorie* is equal to about 4.2 kilojoules. Once again, few people use this unit of measure so we will forgo it also.)

Carbohydrates

Carbohydrates do much more than just fuel our bodies. They also fuel debate. Indeed, there is probably no other area of diabetes management that offers quite the same degree of controversy. In this section we will look at the important issues for you to be aware of, including the pros and cons of low versus higher carbohydrate diets.

Although glucose — a carbohydrate made up of one molecule — gets most of the attention, within our bodies we also have other carbohydrates made up of many molecules, including starches, cellulose, and gums (not the chewing type; although, come to think of it, we can think of more than one occasion when chewing gum has made its way into someone's stomach, but we'll chew on that one some other time).

Carbohydrates are found primarily in things grown in the ground and in dairy foods. Some of the common dietary sources of carbohydrate are bread, potatoes, grains, cereals, rice, dairy products, fruits, and sweet vegetables (such as carrots and squash).

A lot is known about the roles that carbohydrates play in the body:

- Carbohydrates are the primary source of energy for muscles.
- Carbohydrates cause the triglyceride (fat) level to rise in the blood.

✔ Glucose is the carbohydrate that causes the pancreas to release insulin.

✔ When insulin is not present in sufficient amounts or is ineffective, ingesting carbohydrate raises the blood glucose above normal.

✔ Simple sugars (as present in sweets) are not directly harmful (except, perhaps to your teeth) as long as your total number of calories ingested is not excessive.

Consuming "sugar" does *not* cause diabetes. Furthermore, do not let any well-meaning friend or relative tell you that because you have diabetes you cannot eat sugar. You can. Tell them Ian and Alan said so. (We'll leave it up to you if you also want to tell them that you recognize that you have to eat appropriate amounts and types of "sugar.")

A few years ago an 85-year-old man was referred to Ian after having been diagnosed a few months earlier with type 2 diabetes. He was a charming gentleman and clearly was working diligently to maintain his traditionally good health. As they spoke, Ian couldn't help but get the impression that something was bothering his new patient. Finally, because the gentleman was not volunteering anything in this way, Ian asked him point-blank if there might be something on his mind. "Well, Doctor," he said, "I guess I'm just feeling kind of sad that I had my birthday yesterday and everyone got to eat my birthday cake except for me. And it was my favourite, too. Chocolate." Whatever reply this gentleman was expecting, it was clearly not the one that Ian supplied. "Well, sir," Ian said, "I have a prescription I want you to fill. Right after you leave this office I want you to go *not* to the drugstore, but to the *bakery*. Buy the biggest chocolate cake they sell and cut yourself as big a slice as you want. And if anyone tells you that you 'can't eat it because you have diabetes,' you tell them that your diabetes specialist *ordered* you to." The patient left the room literally singing.

Cake is not a four-letter word! If you have diabetes you can eat not only cake, but other sweets too. The point is, nothing is "forbidden," it just has to be consumed in moderation and, most importantly, not at the expense of other, healthier foods that you need. So long as your total number of carbohydrates and calories is appropriate, there is nothing wrong with having occasional treats. Happy birthday!

A greater percentage of Canadians are overweight now than at any other time in our history. This is due primarily to two things. We are not as physically active as we once were. And we are consuming, on average, about 200 calories more per day than we did a generation ago. These extra calories are derived almost exclusively from unneeded carbohydrates in "super-size" soft drinks, "extra-large" candy bars, and excessive consumption of breads, pastries, and the like. Within our bodies, these extra carbohydrates are turned into fat and stored in our fat cells. This ability to store extra calories as fat was great when everyone lived in caves and got little food for prolonged periods of time, but it doesn't fit today's lifestyle, consisting as it does of abundant food (and minimal foraging for it — unless you count hunting through the supermarket aisles).

Because carbohydrate is the food that raises the blood glucose — and high glucose is responsible for many of the complications of diabetes — it is important to consume the proper amount of carbohydrates.

If you are on a 2,000-calorie diet and are consuming 50 percent of your calories as carbohydrate, that would work out to 1,000 calories of carbohydrate per day. Each gram of carbohydrate is 4 calories, so you would be consuming 250 grams of carbohydrate per day. Translating this into foods you know and love, this would work out to about 16 slices of bread (15 grams per slice), 9 cups of cereal (28 grams per cup), or 6 cups of rice (42 grams per cup).

Most people with diabetes do very well on this amount of carbohydrate, but for others a lower percentage works best.

Glycemic index

All carbohydrates are not alike in the degree to which they raise the blood glucose. This fact was recognized some years ago, and a measurement called the glycemic index was created to quantify it. The *glycemic index* (GI) uses white bread as the indicator food and assigns it a value of 100. Another carbohydrate of equal calories is rated according to its ability to raise the blood glucose and assigned a value in comparison to white bread. A food that raises glucose half as much as white bread has a GI of 50, while a food that raises glucose 11/2 times as much has a GI of 150. The point of the index is to select carbohydrates with low GI levels to try to keep the glucose response as low as possible.

Like most things in life, the GI has its supporters and its detractors. Its supporters point out that relying on foods with a low glycemic index has these advantages:

- May help improve blood glucose control
- May help improve lipids (There is often a reduction in levels of triglycerides and LDL cholesterol.)

On the other side of the food fence, GI detractors point out these problems:

- The GI of a carbohydrate may be different when it is eaten alone than when it is part of a mixed meal.
- The GI of a food may differ depending on how it's processed and prepared.
- Some low-GI foods contain a lot of fat.
- Figuring out the GI can be difficult and can lead to confusion.
- Research has not yet proven long-term health benefits of a low-GI diet.

We can think of no better illustration of the controversy regarding the glycemic index than the point that Alan is a supporter and Ian is not yet convinced. Alan would note that he has observed improved glucose control in his patients that follow a low-GI and Ian would point out that a Snickers candy bar rates better on the GI than does a bowl of cornflakes. (We are not making this up!) Is it possible that some people might mistakenly believe this means that candy bars are a healthy food choice? What a disastrous error that would be!

The Canadian Diabetes Association, quite appropriately, feels that the decision to implement a low-glycemic-index diet should be individualized based on a person's particular interest and ability.

Seeing as we do not yet have proof that a low-glycemic-index diet is the way to go, the most prudent course would be to initiate your nutrition therapy with the standard Canadian Diabetes Association guidelines, as you will learn from your dietitian. If you have been working with this meal plan and not succeeding the way you should, speak to your dietitian and your family doctor (and diabetes specialist if you are seeing one) to see if they feel you would benefit by switching to a low-GI diet.

Should you elect to proceed with a low-glycemic-index diet, you can easily make some simple substitutions in your diet, as shown in Table 7-1.

Table 7-1   Simple Diet Substitutions for a Low-GI Diet

High-GI Food	Low-GI Food
Whole meal or white bread	Whole grain bread
Processed breakfast cereal	Unrefined cereals like oats or processed low-GI cereals
Plain cookies and crackers	Cookies made with dried fruits or whole grains like oats
Cakes and muffins	Cakes and muffins made with fruit, oats, and whole grains
Tropical fruits like bananas	Temperate climate fruits like apples and plums
Potatoes	Pasta or legumes
Rice	Basmati or other low-GI rice

Bread and breakfast cereal are major daily sources of carbo-hydrates, so these simple changes can make a major difference in lowering your glycemic index. Foods that are excellent sources of carbohydrate but have a low GI include legumes such as peas or beans, pasta, grains like barley, parboiled rice, and whole grain breads.

The CDA Web site (www.diabetes.ca) lists additional foods based on their GI in a document entitled Glycemic Index Resource.

Carbohydrate Counting

Glucose levels rise after you eat mainly because of the carbo-hydrates in your meal (or snack). Also, in general, the greater the number of grams of carbohydrate, the more your blood glucose level will rise. People who are on an intensified insulin program consisting of frequent injections of short-acting insulin can gauge the amount of insulin to inject based on the number of grams of carbohydrate they are about to ingest.

Fibre

Fibre is the part of the carbohydrate that is not digestible and therefore adds no calories. It is found in most fruits, grains, and vegetables. Fibre comes in two forms:

- ✔ **Soluble fibre:** This form of fibre can dissolve in water and has a lowering effect on blood glucose and fat levels, particularly cholesterol. Soluble fibre gets gooey and sticky when mixed with water. An example is oatmeal.

- ✔ **Insoluble fibre:** This form of fibre cannot dissolve in water and remains in the intestine. It absorbs water and stimulates movement in the intestine. Insoluble fibre also helps prevent constipation and possibly colon cancer. This is the fibre called bulk or roughage. Insoluble fibre does not change much when mixed with water. An example is the skin of an apple.

Before the current trend to refine foods, people ate many sources of carbohydrate that were high in fibre. These were all in plantfoods, such as fruits, vegetables, and grains. Animal foods contain no fibre.

The Canadian Diabetes Association recommends you ingest 25 to 35 grams of fibre daily. Because too much fibre causes diarrhea and gas, you need to increase the fibre level in your diet fairly slowly.

Protein

Unless you are a vegetarian, most of the protein in your diet is derived from the muscle of other animals, such as chicken, turkey, beef, or lamb. The main role that protein has in your diet is to maintain the health of tissues such as your muscles. As it turns out, you do not need to consume much protein in your diet to maintain your current level of muscle. Unlike carbohydrates, proteins do not raise blood glucose levels significantly.

Why proteins do not raise blood glucose

When the protein you ingest passes through the stomach and enters the small intestine, it is broken down into smaller molecules called amino acids. The amino acids are absorbed into the bloodstream and head for the liver, where *some* are converted into glucose (others are used to build new protein). So, although dietary protein can raise glucose, this takes place slowly and is not a major contributor to blood glucose.

Your choice of protein is very important because some protein sources also contain very high quantities of fat while others are relatively fat free. The following lists give you an idea of the fat content of various sources of protein.

About 30 grams (1 oz) of **very lean** meat, fish, or substitutes has 7 grams of protein and 1 gram of fat. Examples are:

- Skinless white-meat chicken or turkey
- Flounder, halibut, or tuna canned in water
- Lobster, shrimp, or clams
- Fat-free cheese

About 30 grams (1 oz) of **lean** meat, fish, or substitutes has 7 grams of protein and 3 grams of fat. Examples are:

- Lean beef, lean pork, lamb, or veal
- Dark-meat chicken without skin or white-meat chicken with skin
- Sardines, salmon, or tuna canned in oil
- Other meats or cheeses with 3 grams of fat per 30 grams (1 oz)

About 30 grams (1 oz) of **medium-fat** meat, fish, or substitutes has 7 grams of protein and 5 grams of fat. Examples are:

- Most beef products
- Regular fat pork, lamb, or veal
- Dark-meat chicken with skin or fried chicken
- Fried fish
- Cheeses with 5 grams of fat per 30 grams (1 oz) such as feta and mozzarella

About 30 grams (1 oz) of **high-fat** meat, fish, or substitutes contains 7 grams of protein and 8 grams of fat. Examples are:

- Pork spareribs or pork sausage
- Bacon
- Regular cheeses such as cheddar and Monterey Jack
- Processed sandwich meats

Depending on whether you choose a high- or low-fat-containing protein source there can be a huge difference in the number of calories. For instance, 30 grams (1 oz) of skinless white meat chicken contains about 40 calories whereas 30 grams (1 oz) of pork spareribs has 100 calories. Because most people eat a minimum of about 120 grams (about 4 ozs) of meat at a meal, they're eating from 160 to 400 calories depending upon the source. That is why it is so important to look carefully at the food you are about to eat; the company your protein source keeps can make the difference between you successfully losing weight or not.

If you are on a 2,000-calorie diet with 20 percent being protein, that would call for 400 calories from protein sources. Because a gram of protein is 4 calories, you could eat 100 grams of protein.

Fat

When we think of fat, we tend to think of the fat we see on a steak or in hamburger meat. But there are actually quite a variety of fats and fat-like substances. Although many of these are unhealthy and to be avoided, some, in fact, help to protect our health. This section looks at these different issues.

Cholesterol is the fat-like substance everyone knows. It has been shown to be a major contributor leading to atherosclerosis (such as coronary artery disease). It is recommended that no more than 300 milligrams a day of fat come from cholesterol. (One large egg has about 210 mg of cholesterol.) Other sources of cholesterol include whole milk and hard cheeses such as Monterey Jack and cheddar.

Most people do not realize the extent to which our bodies (our livers in particular) contribute to our cholesterol levels. In fact, the majority of our body's cholesterol is made by our livers. It is for that reason that so many people with diabetes, even if faithfully following a low-fat diet, end up requiring medication anyhow in order to achieve optimal blood cholesterol levels.

The other kind of fat is triglyceride, which we classify into two groups:

- ✔ **Saturated fat** is the kind of fat that comes from animal sources. The streaks of fat in a steak are saturated fat. Butter, bacon, cream, and cream cheese are other examples of foods rich in saturated fat. Eating a lot of saturated fat can make your bad (LDL) cholesterol level go up. And that is not a good thing.

- ✔ **Unsaturated fat** comes from vegetable sources such as olive oil, canola oil, and margarine. It comes in several forms:

   - • **Monounsaturated fat** does not raise cholesterol. Avocado, olive oil, and canola oil are examples. The oil in nuts such as almonds and peanuts is also monounsaturated.

> • **Polyunsaturated fat** does not raise cholesterol but can lead to a reduction in HDL cholesterol (this is the "good" cholesterol). Examples of polyunsaturated fats are soft fats and oils such as corn oil, mayonnaise, and margarine. Polyunsaturated fats should be less than 10 percent of your total calorie intake.

You may have read recently about "trans" fatty acids. Trans fatty acids also raise LDL levels. They are formed when vegetable oil goes through a process of hydrogenation during the manufacture of many commercially baked goods such as cookies, cakes, potato chips, and some types of margarines.

Saturated and trans fatty acids combined should be restricted to less than 10 percent of your calorie intake.

Lest you think that everything with the word *fat* in it is bad, here is some good news about fat. Some fats are actually good for you. There is mounting evidence that a fat called *omega-3 fatty acids* can help protect you from atherosclerosis. These acids are found in certain fish such as salmon, tuna, mackerel, and trout. Omega-3 fatty acids also help reduce blood pressure and protect against the formation of blood clots in the coronary arteries (thus reducing the likelihood of your getting a heart attack). It is recommended that you eat fish rich in omega-3 fatty acids at least once (better still, two or three times) per week. If you don't like fish, we can't help but think that it must mean you have never tasted salmon cooked on a barbecue or in a dishwasher. (True story: Ian's mom makes marvellous "dishwasher salmon," and no, the fish does not swim around in the water; it is wrapped in tinfoil and put through the entire wash and dry cycle — without soap! Readers can find a variety of dishwasher salmon recipes on the Internet.)

If we go back to your hypothetical 2,000-calorie diet — lest you slowly starve while waiting for us to figure out how much fat to feed you so that you get your final 600 calories — fat has 9 calories per gram, so you can eat about 67 grams of fat daily. Seeing as you may have consumed much of this with your protein source, you may not have much fat left to add.

Vitamins, minerals, and water

Your nutrition plan must contain sufficient vitamins and minerals, but the amount you need may be less than you think. If you eat a balanced diet that comes from the various food groups, you will generally get enough vitamins for your daily needs. Table 7-2 lists the vitamins and their food sources.

Table 7-2	Vitamins You Need	
Vitamin	*Function*	*Food Source*
Vitamin A	Needed for healthy skin and bones	Milk and green vegetables
Vitamin B1 (thiamine)	Converts carbohydrates into energy	Meat and whole grain cereals
Vitamin B2 (riboflavin)	Needed to use food properly	Milk, cheese, fish, and green vegetables
Vitamin B6 (pyridoxine)	Needed for growth	Liver, yeast, and many other foods
Vitamin B12	Keeps the red blood cells and the nervous system healthy	Animal foods (for example, meat)
Folic acid (also called folate)	Keeps the red blood cells healthy	Green vegetables
Niacin	Helps maintain healthy metabolism	Lean meat, fish, nuts, and legumes
Vitamin C	Helps maintain supportive tissues	Fruit and potatoes
Vitamin D	Helps with absorption of calcium	Dairy products and is made in the skin when exposed to sunlight
Vitamin E	Helps maintain cells	Vegetable oils and whole grain cereals
Vitamin K	Needed for proper clotting of the blood	Green, leafy vegetables

As you look through the vitamins in Table 7-2, you can see that most of them are readily available in the foods you eat every day. In certain situations, such as if you are pregnant or breastfeeding, elderly, a strict vegetarian, or on a very low calorie diet, you should take a multivitamin daily. (In pregnancy you should also take a folic acid supplement.)

Although Canadians spend millions upon millions of dollars each year on vitamin supplements, these supplements are seldom helpful (except for the people selling them!). Our clever bodies are quite adept at knowing when we have enough vitamins in our system, and when you take in extra quantities you either store them in your fat or you have very expensive urine. By way of example, recent medical studies showed that taking extra vitamin E provided no additional health value. Yet until those studies were published, tens of millions of dollars (perhaps hundreds of millions) was being spent each year in North America on vitamin E supplements. We would strongly recommend that if you have good nutrition (and thereby will get all the vitamins you need), you take the money you might be spending on vitamin supplements and donate it to your favourite charity.

Not only are routine vitamin supplements not necessary, but a recent study found that Vitamin E supplements may actually be harmful (the study found a higher risk of heart failure in people taking Vitamin E supplements). "Megadoses" of certain vitamins are a particular concern. For example, high doses of vitamin A can lead to liver damage and too much Vitamin D can cause vomiting and muscle weakness.

Minerals are also key ingredients of a healthy diet. Most are needed in tiny amounts, easily consumed from a balanced diet. These are the main minerals you should know:

- ✔ **Calcium:** We need calcium primarily to maintain strong bones. Insufficient calcium intake can be a factor in developing osteoporosis. Milk and other dairy products provide plenty of calcium. It is important to ingest between 1,000 and 1,500 milligrams of calcium per day. If you are not consuming enough calcium in your diet, you should take calcium supplements. If you are growing up (adolescents) or out (pregnant women) this also applies.

Before you start taking calcium supplements it is important to check with your physician to make sure you are not taking any other medicine or do not have any other health problem that could lead to abnormally high blood calcium levels.

✔ **Chromium:** We require chromium for certain internal chemical reactions to take place normally. In areas of the world where there is a severe deficiency of chromium in the diet, people are more likely to develop diabetes. Regrettably, people in areas of the world where we get perfectly adequate quantities of chromium in our diets (this includes Canada) have been inundated with pseudo-scientific and misleading claims that taking chromium supplements will either reduce your blood glucose levels or cure your diabetes. We have no convincing evidence of the former and as for the latter, it is simply false. Once again, the only people benefitting from this promotion are the people selling the products.

✔ **Iodine:** Iodine is necessary for our thyroid glands to work normally. You may have noticed that boxes of salt in Canada are labelled "Iodized." Because of this iodine supplementation, Canadians do not develop iodine deficiency (even if you never add salt to your food).

✔ **Iron:** We require iron to make red blood cells. A lack of iron leads to anemia. Most of our iron intake comes from consumption of red meat. Menstruating women are prone to iron deficiency (menstrual blood is rich in iron) and often will require iron supplementation. Vegetarians also often require iron supplements.

✔ **Magnesium:** Our bodies use magnesium to allow a number of different chemical reactions to occur. Magnesium deficiency can lead to problems with the heart's electrical system. Magnesium deficiency is very seldom a problem and routine supplements are unnecessary.

✔ **Phosphorous:** Phosphorous in our bodies contributes to the maintenance of strong bones. We get ample phosphorous in our diets and routine supplements are not required.

✔ **Sodium:** Getting sufficient quantities of sodium ("salt") in Canadian diets is not a problem. Quite the opposite. We uniformly consume excess quantities. Sodium is present in many of the foods we eat — particularly in processed foods such as prepared meats and some cheeses, as well as packaged snack foods such as pretzels and potato chips. You may be surprised to know that Canadians consume an astounding 20 times more sodium per day than we need. This may be a factor leading to high blood pressure. You would be wise to avoid adding salt to your food, and if you have high blood pressure, make a point of buying foods that are low in salt to begin with.

✔ **Cobalt, Tin, and Zinc:** These minerals are rarely lacking in the human diet and supplements are unnecessary.

Although we have saved our discussion about water to last, it is by no means the least important. Your body is made up of 60 percent or more water. All the nutrients in the body are dissolved in water. You can live without food for some time, but you will not last long without water. Water can help to give a feeling of fullness that reduces appetite. You should make a point of drinking at least 1^{1}/$_{2}$ litres (50 oz) of water per day.

A whole industry has developed based on the assumption that tap water is not as healthy for you as bottled water. There is, in fact, a *huge* difference between tap water and bottled water. Last time we checked, this difference was a penny or two compared to about a dollar. If you want to drink bottled water because you prefer the taste, go for it. If you are drinking bottled water because you think it is healthier, we would suggest that you take the dollar a day you plan on spending and put it toward purchasing some new running shoes.

Artificial and sugar alcohol sweeteners

Unrestricted consumption of sugars does not fit with good diabetes management (or, of course, with good health in general). And since there are limits on how much sugar we should consume, artificial sweeteners have a role to play. Of the artificial sweeteners in common use, aspartame

(NutraSweet) is the best known. In the amounts commonly used, aspartame provides virtually no calories, yet provides abundant sweetness. In fact, aspartame is 200 times sweeter than sucrose (table sugar). Aspartame has been the subject of many Internet rumours detailing its dangers. These are false. The truth of the matter is that aspartame is completely safe unless you have a rare genetic disease called PKU. The equal truth is that despite common use of aspartame in our society, we as a population are getting larger and larger, not smaller and smaller.

Other approved artificial sweeteners in Canada are saccharin (Sweet'n Low), cyclamate (sucaryl; this is the sweetener used in Sugar Twin), sucralose (Splenda), and acesuflame potassium (Sunett). These are safe for use if you have diabetes — unless you are pregnant or breastfeeding, in which case you should not consume saccharin or cyclamate.

Sugar alcohols (maltitol, mannitol, sorbitol, isomalt, and xylitol) are another type of sweetener. They are not artificial. They do provide calories and can affect your blood glucose levels to a degree. Examples of products that may contain sugar alcohols are chewing gum, hard candies, some jams, and syrups. Consumption of more than 10 grams per day of sugar alcohols can cause abdominal cramping and diarrhea.

Alcohol

Alcohol is a substance that has calories but no particular nutritional value. It has, however, been shown that a moderate amount (a drink or two per day) may reduce your risk of a heart attack.

If you like to have a drink, it is reasonable that you continue so long as you limit yourself to no more than two drinks per day if you are a man, and one drink per day if you are a woman. If you do not normally drink, do not start just because you are at possible risk of developing heart disease down the road. And, of course, if you are pregnant, you should not drink any alcohol at all.

Having two drinks per day is *not* the same as quaffing 14 cold ones on a Saturday evening while you watch *Hockey Night in Canada*. Even if the game goes into overtime.

Because alcohol has calories, you must account for the alcohol you drink in your diet. Depending on the strength of the individual product, 350 millilitres (12 oz) of beer, 150 millilitres (5 oz) of wine, and 45 millilitres (11/2 oz) of hard liquor all have similar quantities of alcohol.

Despite what many people think, drinking beer or wine is not "better for you" than drinking hard liquor. To your liver they all taste the same.

Apart from the consequences of the calories it provides, there are several other important points about alcohol to keep in mind:

- ✔ Alcohol — especially if taken without food — can cause low blood glucose if you are on insulin or some forms of oral hypoglycemic agent therapy. It does this by reducing your liver's ability to produce glucose. You can lessen this risk by making sure you eat some food when you are drinking alcohol.

- ✔ Alcohol reduces your awareness of symptoms of low blood glucose and as a result, makes you less likely to take appropriate corrective action.

- ✔ Alcohol can interact with some medicines called sulfony-lurea oral hypoglycemic agents and cause a variety of unpleasant symptoms including nausea and flushing (even if you are not inebriated).

- ✔ If you are on insulin or certain medicines that stimulate insulin production, drinking alcohol 2 or 3 hours after your supper can result in hypoglycemia occurring the next morning after breakfast.

The Atkins Diet

There is seldom a shortage of controversy over diets, especially when it comes to the diet recommended by the late Dr. Robert Atkins.

The Atkins diet recommends the consumption of very small amounts of carbohydrate and substantial quantities of protein and fat.

The main potential advantages of this diet:

- ✔ Many people find it allows them to lose weight when other diets have not.

- ✔ Blood glucose control often improves.

The main potential disadvantages of this diet:

- ✔ The weight that is lost is often regained.

- ✔ People commonly develop hair loss.

- ✔ Most people do not adhere to this diet for very long (as is the case with all diets that are very restrictive, people tire of them).

- ✔ Many healthy foods are potentially eliminated from the diet.

- ✔ There is some evidence that a high-protein diet can lead to worrisome problems including calcium loss from the bones (which could potentially lead to osteoporosis), kidney stones, an increase in LDL ("bad") cholesterol, dizziness, and, though not dangerous, problematic constipation and fatigue.

Research has also found that the weight loss that occurs with the Atkins diet is due primarily to lower calorie intake; the fact that fewer carbohydrates are ingested is of less importance.

Suffice to say, there are advocates, fans, and even zealots on both sides of the Atkins fence. Although the jury is out, history shows that diets that advocate an extreme diet management approach have invariably failed because people get tired of the severe restrictions they contain and eventually abandon them. How else to explain the fact that many (perhaps most by now) homes in Canada have so many different diet books, each book having its own particular bent and often saying things opposite to the book sitting next to it on the bookshelf?

Weighty Issues

In Chapter 3 we discuss the various ways you can determine whether you are overweight. If you are, then you are in good company. Millions of Canadians are also overweight, as are the great majority of people with type 2 diabetes. But (we love being able to add a "but" here) we are now going to work our hardest at improving your health, and one of the most important steps is to, well, take steps.

As it turns out, you will soon see the benefits of weight loss, even when you have lost relatively little weight. Blood glucose falls rapidly. Blood pressure declines. Bad (LDL) cholesterol falls as do fats (triglycerides), and good cholesterol (HDL) rises. How neat is that! We suspect that if we were to market a drug that had all these attributes it would be considered a "wonder drug."

You should aim to lose 1 to 2 kilograms (2 to 4 lbs) per month, 5 to 10 percent of your initial body weight over 6 months. Losing weight faster than that increases the likelihood that you will regain it. You should try to burn off 500 calories more per day than you ingest. (To calculate what this requires, have a look at the calorie content of carbohydrates, proteins, and fats earlier in this chapter.) Although you will need to reduce your intake of carbohydrate, you should make sure you consume at least 100 grams of carbohydrate per day. Ingesting less than that will lead to loss of muscle tissue and can affect your fluid balance. Also, if you eat lots of high-fibre foods you will find that you won't feel as hungry.

At the risk of sounding like a late-night TV commercial, when it comes to the benefits of weight loss, "you get all this and more." More? Yes, more. Weight loss will also accomplish the following:

- ✔ Allow blood pressure and oral hypoglycemic agent medications to work more effectively
- ✔ Improve your sense of well-being
- ✔ Make you feel more energetic and more inclined to exercise
- ✔ Increase your life expectancy

Weight reduction is difficult for many reasons, but perhaps foremost among these is the immense challenge of trying to change lifestyle patterns and habits that you may have lived with for decades. No one should ever tell you that the changes you are being asked to make are easy. They are not easy. In fact, for most people they are downright difficult. But they can be done. And if you have initial success only to then revert back to old habits, that does not mean all is lost. Just pick up where you left off and try again.

Half a kilogram (about a pound) of fat contains 3,500 calories. Therefore, in order to lose this much fat, you must eat 3,500 calories less than you need or you must burn off these calories by exercising. Often the best strategy is to combine reduced calorie intake with increased calorie expenditure. So grab your walking shoes and bypass the fridge as you head for the door for your new, daily walk.

Surgery for weight loss

Surgery is sometimes used in the most severe and resistant cases of obesity (BMI 35 or greater; see the chart in Chapter 3). For select individuals it can be a very effective form of therapy, with multiple health benefits including improved glucose control.

The most effective surgical treatment for obesity is the Roux-en-Y gastric bypass operation, where the stomach is stapled to create a small pouch. A section of the small intestine is attached to the pouch so that food passes through very little of the small intestine, reducing calorie and nutrient absorption. Because the pouch is small, you tend to eat less.

As you might imagine, surgery — any surgery — is not to be undertaken lightly. (There is an old expression that "minor surgery" is surgery that someone else has.) Potential drawbacks include direct complications from the procedure (wound breakdown, infection, and so on) and more remote complications (including deficiency of certain vitamins and minerals due to inadequate absorption, anemia, diarrhea, and hypoglycemia).

Behaviour modification

We've already talked about the importance of lifestyle change to help reduce your weight and enhance your health. And we've also already mentioned just how difficult changing long-standing eaten patterns can be. Here are some tips you may find helpful in your quest to adjust your eating habits:

- Eat at set times.

- Eat your food in a single place.

- Slow down your eating.

- Put your cutlery down between mouthfuls.

- Don't put more food in your mouth before you have finished your last bite.

- Concentrate on the taste of each mouthful before you swallow.

- Every few minutes, pause and ask yourself if you are still hungry.

- Don't finish every morsel on your plate. There is nothing wrong with leaving some behind.

- After the food has been served, remove the serving dishes and bread basket from the table.

- Don't keep high-calorie snacks visible in the kitchen or elsewhere in the house. Better yet, don't keep them in the house at all.

- Remember that seemingly innocent things like salad dressings can be very rich in calories.

- Add bulk to your food (adding vegetable to pasta for example). Hunger is often satisfied by increasing the volume of food even if the number of calories is reduced.

- Avoid "impulse buying" when doing your groceries. Bring a shopping list and walk the aisles specifically looking for the items you have written down rather than just wandering from aisle to aisle.

- Get a 5-kilogram weight and carry it around for a while to appreciate the importance of a loss of even that little.

✔ Incorporate regular exercise into your weight-loss strategy.

✔ Most important of all, remember that there is no rush. As we say earlier, trying to lose weight too rapidly will make it more likely that you will regain the weight later.

As you go about the difficult task of losing weight and keeping it off, remember to seek the help of those around you. A loving partner provides great help through the roughest days.

Notes

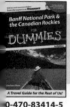

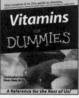
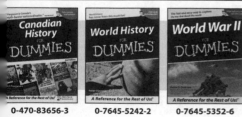

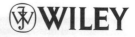

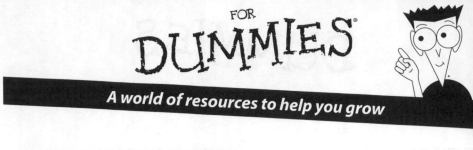

FOR DUMMIES®

A world of resources to help you grow

COMPUTERS, INTERNET & DIGITAL MEDIA

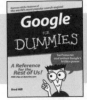

Google For Dummies
0-7645-4420-9

eBay For Dummies
0-7645-5654-1

Digital Photography For Dummies
0-7645-9802-3

Also available:

CD and DVD Recorded For Dummies 2/e
(0-7645-5956-7)

Genealogy Online For Dummies 4/e
(0-7645-5964-8)

PCs For Dummies 10/e
(0-7645-8958-X)

Internet For Dummies 10/e
(0-7645-8996-2)

Windows XP For Dummies 2/e
(0-7645-7326-8)

PERSONAL FINANCE & BUSINESS

Investing For Canadians For Dummies
1-8944-1300-8

Buying and Selling a Home For Canadians For Dummies
0-470-83320-3

Personal Finance For Canadians For Dummies
1-894413-29-6

Also available:

Accounting For Dummies 3/e
(0-7645-7836-7)

Canadian Small Business Kit For Dummies
(1-894413-04-0)

Stock Investing For Canadians For Dummies
(0-470-83342-4)

Wills & Estates For Canadians For Dummies
(1-894413-17-2)

FITNESS, HOBBIES & PETS

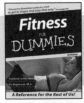

Fitness For Dummies
0-7645-5167-1

Auto Repair For Dummies
0-7645-5089-6

Guitar For Dummies
0-7645-9904-6

Also available:

Cats For Dummies 2/e
(0-7645-5275-9)

Chess For Dummies 2/e
(0-7645-8404-9)

Dog Training For Dummies
(0-7645-5286-4)

Knitting For Dummies
(0-7645-5395-X)

Bridge For Dummies
(0-7645-5015-2)

Piano For Dummies
(0-7645-5105-1)

Pilates For Dummies
(0-7645-5397-6)

Sudoku For Dummies
(0-470-01892-5)

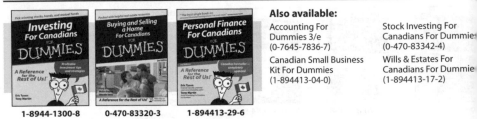

Available wherever books are sold. Go to www.dummies.com or call 1-877-762-2974 to order direct

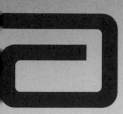

The Friends for Life Program*

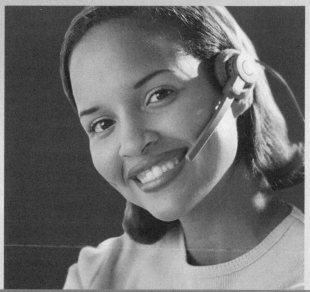

Friends for Life

Abbott Diabetes Care monitors come with an extensive Customer Care Program

- Customer Care team available 24 hours a day, 7 days a week
- Free educational support materials available through Customer Care centre
- Comprehensive expert training and technical advice provided by our Customer Care team
- Free lifetime monitor upgrades*

Customer Care Centre 1 888 519-6890

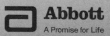

Abbott

A Promise for Life